Marina Andrews becai
Sunday Express in 1962, and joined *Vogue* as Diet Columnist several years later. During the last fifteen years she has freelanced for most of the women's magazines in Britain and the Far East. She has also worked on various Health and Fitness television series and lectured extensively in schools, colleges and women's groups in this country and abroad.

In 1969 she was appointed Managing Director of Town & Country Health Salons Ltd, where she runs the Health and Beauty School. On a daily basis she is consulted on nutrition and general health problems. Her clientele come from all walks of life, and have included royalty, Hollywood stars, doctors and members of the House of Lords. At present she is engaged in health projects for the Middle East and Nigeria.

She is the author of four previous cookery books.

Sunday Express Diet Book

MARINA ANDREWS

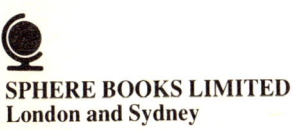

SPHERE BOOKS LIMITED
London and Sydney

First published in Great Britain by
Sphere Books Ltd, 1986
30–32 Gray's Inn Road, London WC1X 8JL
Copyright © Marina Andrews, 1986

For my husband

TRADE
MARK

This book is sold subject to the condition that
it shall not, by way of trade or otherwise, be lent,
re-sold, hired out or otherwise circulated without
the publisher's prior consent in any form of
binding or cover other than that in which it is
published and without a similar condition
including this condition being imposed on the
subsequent purchaser.

Set in Linotron Trump 9/10

Printed and bound in Great Britain by
Cox & Wyman Ltd, Reading

Contents

Introduction   xi

ONE-DAY DIETS
Fruit and Nut Salad Diet   2
Grapefruit and Champagne Diet   3
Inner Cleanliness Diet   4
Super Quick Diet   5
Raisin and Cheese Diet   6
World's Cheapest Diet   7
Vitality Diet   8

TWO-DAY DIETS
Avocado Diet   10
Bovril Diet   12
Desperate Diet   13
Orange and Grapefruit Diet   14
Last Minute Diet   16
Panic Stations Diet   17
Strawberry Diet   18

THREE-DAY DIETS
Cheese and Tomato Diet   22
Melon Diet   24
New Year Diet   26
Quickie Fruit Diet   28
Summer Diet   29
Tantalising Diet   30
Simple Banana Diet   31

FOUR-DAY DIETS
Apple and Cheese Diet   34

vi *Sunday Express Diet Book*

Ayram Health Diet	36
Cheese Diet	38
Honey, Milk and Almond Diet	39
Liberal Diet	40
Orange Cocktail and Cheese Diet	41
Winter Vitamin Cup Diet	42

ONE-WEEK DIETS

Easy Diet	44
Eight Meals a Day Diet	48
Final Diet	50
Fruit and Vegetable Alternating Diet	52
Fruits of Summer Diet	54
Gourmet Diet	56
Super Diet	61

TWO-WEEK DIETS

Yoghurt Diet	64
Alternating Diet	66
Wonder Diet	68
Dorothy's Onion Diet	70
Painless Diet	72
Revitalising Diet	74
Booster Diet	76

THREE-WEEK DIETS

Monday to Friday Diet	80
Try me Diet	84
Sherry Diet	86
Three by Three Diet	88
My High Fibre Diet	90
Day by Day Diet	93
Winter Flab Diet	94

FOUR-WEEK DIETS

Hungry Man's Diet	98
Monday to Sunday Diet	103
Secretary's Diet	106
Slimmer's Lunch Plan Diet	111
Weekends Only Diet	115
Strawberry Banana and Yogurt Diet	116
Incentive Diet	118

TWO-MONTH DIETS
Town and Country Diet 124
Total Diet 129
Miss Great Britain Diet 132
I Love to Eat Diet 135

Sunday Express Diet Book

Introduction

A question I am often asked by my clients, colleagues and friends is: 'How do you manage to write so many different diets?' The answer to that is very simple:
a) it has been a life-long job (25 years) consulting with people about their daily eating habits, thereby giving me a first-class understanding of the needs and weaknesses of weight gains and losses;
b) I have always been very interested in food as a subject, not just as a means of living but as a diversity which has to be created, changed and adapted to the mood and high technology of present-day living, as well as the good health of the consumer; and
c) as a regular diet columnist with the *Sunday Express* (23 years) I have to keep my readers stimulated!

To introduce *you* to my way of dieting I have selected 60 of my favourite, well-tried and tested slimming regimes. The diets range from One-Day Inner Cleanliness routines to a Two-Months Complete Eating Plan. There are 7 diets to choose from in each group – hopefully catering to all likes and dislikes – together with a note of the average weight loss that can be achieved during the period of the diet. In the two-month range there is a choice of four different diets with something to suit the whole family, including children.

Which diet is right for you will depend very much upon:
1) how overweight you are to start with, and
2) the combination of foods and their appeal to your tastes.
These are two very important points, especially the foods which are to be eaten, because if they do not appeal to the dieter then he or she is not going to stay on the diet. Far too many diets stipulate foods that are boring or expensive or simply lacking in imagination; others are complicated or difficult and time-consuming in preparation – again failing to retain the discipline of the would-be dieter. My own proven statistics have shown that my diets do work where others

have failed, in showing both good weight loss and maintenance of that loss.

This latter point is a vitally important part of all slimming and health regimes. How to keep weight off once the desired loss has been achieved! My method is very simple. For example, if you followed one of my three-week or four-week diets and lost, say, one stone (the maximum you wanted to lose), then resumed normal but careful eating habits and perhaps at a wedding or party you over-indulged and found that you had regained, say, 3 lb., act immediately, don't delay, put yourself back on to one of my one-day or two-day diets, which show immediate weight loss. It is so easy for a 3 lb. gain to become 6 lb. if left for a period of, say, 2 weeks. Another excellent maintenance programme is to follow one of my one-day diets in every 7 or 8 days. This way, prevention is far better than cure!

Here are just a few quotes from letters I have received:

> I am the fattest girl in my class and everyone laughs at me, and they call me Bub. After the first two weeks of the diet I found it much easier – I used to weigh 70 kilos, now my weight in just two months is down to 55 kilos. I wish you could see how many friends I have now.
> M FLORENCE, 14-yr-old schoolgirl.

> I am 64 yrs. old and have suffered for the past thirteen years with Diverticulitis. My doctor put me on medication but after following your diet not only did I lose the weight I wanted, but I have stopped taking my medication as my condition has improved 100 pc.
> MRS J M YAFT, Oswestry, Salop

> I have found the diet most satisfying with no ill effects. My weight loss is already 4 lb. in 4 days. My husband is a Consultant Physician and highly approves of the diet, wishing he had the tenacity to stick to it as well!
> A PORTNOY, Manchester

> Thanks to your marvellous diet, I have got down lower than I have since when I was 24 and weighed 9 st. 9 lb., and now at 52 I weighed 11st. 10 lb. I did it slowly every

other weekend and in roughly three months I had lost one stone. I have adapted the diet slightly and still keep to it at weekends. My results have been watched by all my friends, I even sent a copy of the diet to Malta. You have made a lot of people happy and healthier.

MRS M EDWARDS, Northants

I lost 2 stone following the diet three days out of each week and am now the weight I was before having my two children – it was so simple. I've achieved such spectacular loss of inches from 35–30–39 to 34–26–36. Loads of my friends are following the diet too. My husband took me out and treated me to a whole new spring wardrobe and the ladies in the boutique even asked for a copy of THE DIET!

C WILLIAMS, Bucks

Just to tell you that my husband tried the diet for seven days and lost 12½ lb. He is now on it one day a week with good results. One of our receptionists gave it to her two daughters – one lost 5 lb. the other 6 lb. in five days. It is the simplest diet I have yet found and have advised several patients about it.

DR M C, Gateshead, Tyne & Wear

Just to write and say how much my husband and I are enjoying your diet. I feel wonderfully alert – lively and full of energy – what a wonderful way to lose weight and be healthy.

H ASH, London NW11

Congratulations on your diet. I weighed 18½ stone and now I am under 16 stone. Just thought you'd like to know how successful it can be.

PETER C, Blackheath, SE3

I feel I must write and thank you for your marvellous diet. For the first time in many years I have lost 5 lb. in as many days, I feel wonderful. I had fluid on the lungs and was not able to exercise so put on weight. I am now hopeful. Thank you again. P.S. My age is 72.

J OLIVER, Lancing, Sussex

I read with scepticism your diet. I always viewed all diets with suspicion, mainly due to the incredible difficulty in trying to maintain diets. However your diet seemed so simple my wife and I decided to try it and have to admit it was just as successful as you said it would be. We both lost an average of 2 lb. a day over 4–5 days. Neither of us felt tired. The diet was so appetising.

R HELLEWELL, London W1

As you can see by the quotes from the many letters I receive, men, women and children have benefited from my diets, whether they are short-term or long-term. Some have made their own adaptations to suit their lifestyle, but what stands out in most of the letters I have received is that my diets are easy and quick to show results, and that is what all dieters want. No one is perfect, everyone has a weakness – the challenge is to try to overcome the weakness and, by so doing, life is more fun.

One-Day Diets

How and why are one-day diets effective? Well, the easiest way to answer this is to describe a one-day diet as a short 'nap' for the abdomen. It is a period of rest and is the ideal diet if time is short or you need to lose a couple of pounds very quickly. As it is only for one day, there is not a great deal of inconvenience, and probably no one will even notice that you are on a diet.

FRUIT AND NUT SALAD DIET
(average weight loss 3 lb. in one day)

This diet consists of a most delicious combination of fresh fruit and peanuts, which you eat throughout the day in small portions whenever you feel hungry. The drink can also be used as a meal substitute on days when you are not following a rigid diet regime.

For one day's supply of the fruit and nut salad you will need:

5 large oranges
2 fresh grapefruit
6 prunes which have been soaked, or you could use tinned ones
4–5 large strawberries
1 lemon
1 teaspoon undiluted orange squash
1 tablespoon salted peanuts

Method
Peel and segment the oranges and grapefruit, stone and chop the prunes, and cut the strawberries in half. Then put all the ingredients into a large bowl. Add the juice of 1 fresh lemon plus 1 teaspoon of undiluted orange squash. Toss all ingredients well together and finally add 1 heaped tablespoon of salted peanuts. Keep cool in the fridge and eat in small portions throughout the day whenever you feel hungry.

Plus You may have up to 5 glasses of bottled mineral water or herbal tea

GRAPEFRUIT AND CHAMPAGNE DIET
(average weight loss 2½ lb. in one day)

This unusual diet was passed on to me by a very good friend in Paris, who said it never failed to work for her whenever she needed to lose a couple of pounds quickly. I would like to suggest that this is really a stay-at-home diet with as little activity as possible.

BREAKFAST (8–9 AM)
1 whole grapefruit with 1 teaspoon sugar
1 small cup of black coffee (no sugar or milk is to be added, but you may use an artificial sweetener)

11 AM
1 small wine glass of chilled champagne

LUNCH (12–1.30 PM)
1 whole grapefruit with 1 teaspoon sugar
1 small wine glass of chilled champagne

2.30 PM
1 small wine glass of chilled champagne

3.30 PM
½ grapefruit with ½ teaspoon sugar

5.30 PM
1 small wine glass of chilled champagne

6.30 PM
½ grapefruit with ½ teaspoon sugar

7.30 PM
1 small wine glass of chilled champagne

DINNER (8.30 PM)
1 whole grapefruit with 1 teaspoon sugar
1 small wine glass of chilled champagne

Before retiring, take 1 final wine glass of chilled champagne and I think you will find, as I did, that the number of glasses of champagne permitted throughout the day will be adequately contained in the one bottle.

INNER CLEANLINESS DIET
(average weight loss 3 lb. in one day)

This one-day diet is taken in the form of a health drink with added protein and, in addition to aiding weight loss, you will feel healthier and better for it.

For one day's supply of the health drink you will need:

1 lb. (450 g) fresh tomatoes, peeled and quartered. A 15 oz. (425 g) can of tomatoes will do if fresh ones are unobtainable.
2 oz. (50 g) cheese, coarsely grated
½ raw onion, quartered
1 stick of celery
½ green pepper, washed and deseeded
salt and black pepper to taste
Evian water to dilute

Method
Put all the ingredients into a liquidiser and mix until smooth. Season to taste and add bottled mineral water until required consistency is achieved.

This should make eight small glasses of liquid food. One glass is to be taken every two hours throughout the day.

SUPER QUICK DIET
(average weight loss 3 lb. in one day)

The Super Quick Diet is very simple, and consists of a delicious fruit and vegetable salad which is eaten throughout the day in place of normal meals. It is satisfying even to the heartiest of appetites.

BREAKFAST
1 bowl of salad, a day's supply for 2 persons (halve the quantity for 1 person) consisting of 1 small melon, 1½ cucumbers and 6 average-sized tomatoes, to be prepared as follows:

First peel and dice the cucumber. Next, peel, deseed and dice the melon. Skin, deseed and dice the tomatoes. Place all the ingredients in a large bowl, and add a dressing made with 1 tablespoon of white wine vinegar, 1 tablespoon of oil, pepper and garlic salt to taste. Pour over the salad and toss. Store the salad in the bottom of the refrigerator until you are ready to eat it.

Plus 1 small glass of fruit juice
1 crispbread, topped with a very thin slice of hard cheese such as Cheddar, Edam or Gouda
1 small cup of tea with lemon, but no sugar

LUNCH
1 bowl of salad, as before
1 plain yoghurt
1 small cup of tea with lemon, but no sugar

DINNER
1 small glass of fruit juice
1 bowl of salad, as before
1 crispbread, topped with 1 heaped tablespoon of cottage cheese
1 small cup of tea with lemon, but no sugar

RAISIN AND CHEESE DIET
(average weight loss 3 lb. in one day)

This delicious diet is ideal for busy people since no cooking is required. Try to choose a different cheese with each meal to add variety.

BREAKFAST
Juice of 1 fresh orange or lemon, topped up with a little hot water
1 cup of black coffee or tea with lemon, but no sugar or milk
2 oz. (50 g) cheese of your choice
1 handful raisins

MID-MORNING
1 cup of black coffee or tea with lemon, but no sugar or milk

LUNCH
Cheese and raisin bowl made as follows:

Finely chop up 3 or 4 fresh sprigs of parsley. Cube 2 oz. (50 g) cheese of your choice, plus 1 handful of raisins, plus a small wedge of lemon. Put the cheese into a small fruit dish, mix with the raisins, squeeze the juice over from the lemon. Add chopped parsley, mix together and it is now ready to eat. And it is absolutely delicious.

Plus 1 cup of tea with lemon, but no sugar or milk

TEA-TIME
1 cup of tea with lemon, but no sugar or milk

DINNER
2 oz. (50 g) cheese of your choice
1 handful of raisins
1 cup of black coffee or tea with lemon, but no sugar or milk

All drinks must be taken without sugar, but if necessary an artificial sweetener is allowed. The handful of raisins should be as many as you can hold in one generously cupped hand.

WORLD'S CHEAPEST DIET
(average weight loss 3 lb. in one day)

This diet is from a Scandinavian Health Clinic and, not only do you lose weight, but it is an ideal health treatment for the skin, especially for conditions like eczema. Swedish doctors highly recommended it at the Health Clinic.

The diet itself is so simple that anyone could try it. You simply drink up to two pints (1150 ml) of water a day. The water is derived by boiling about 2 lb. (900 g) of well-scrubbed, unpeeled, fresh potatoes in approximately 2½ pints (1425 ml) of water for about 4–5 minutes, by which time all the necessary goodness will have been extracted into the water. The water is then allowed to cool and finely chopped fresh parsley or mint can be added before drinking it. The 2½ pints (1425 ml) should be measured out to last a day, during which time nothing else should be consumed at all.

I suggest you give the diet a try for just twenty-four hours. This cannot do you any harm and you will certainly feel much better – if not lighter – for it. If you feel you can tackle it for two whole days, then good luck.

VITALITY DIET
(average weight loss 3 lb. in one day)

This is a booster diet which is always helpful if you are feeling depressed about your weight. It helps to clear the system and replenish it with new-found energy. The diet is also full of essential vitamins and goodness, and is made up in the form of a vitality cup which is taken throughout the day in place of normal meals.

For one day's supply of the vitality cup, you will need:

1½ pints (850 ml) milk
1 small carton of natural yoghurt
½ pint (275 ml) tomato juice
2 level teaspoons finely chopped parsley
2 teaspoons Worcestershire sauce
1 fresh egg
1 level teaspoon powdered yeast
1 dessertspoon sherry

Method
First, beat the egg till frothy, then add the yeast, yoghurt and the rest of the ingredients. If you have a liquidiser, so much the better. Keep the mixture in a large jug in the bottom of the refrigerator, and drink in small quantities throughout the day whenever you feel hungry, making sure to give it a good stir before you drink it.

Two-Day Diets

Two-day diets are ideal for a 'weekend break' from eating and drinking, especially if you can persuade a friend to join you. This makes the diet even more pleasant and you could compete with each other as to who loses the most weight. If it is not possible to follow the diet on the Saturday or Sunday, try Monday and Friday – it does not have to be two consecutive days – and that will allow you to get rid of any excess pounds incurred over the previous weekend or to prepare you for the onslaught of a heavy weekend's eating.

AVOCADO DIET
(average weight loss 3 lb. in two days)

The avocado is a highly nutritious but under-rated slimming food; with approximately only 132 calories per half, it contains eleven vitamins and seventeen minerals and over two per cent protein oil. To aid weight loss, why not try my special Avocado diet?

BREAKFAST
½ avocado, eaten from the shell. Remove the stone and fill with 2 tablespoons cottage cheese. Add a squeeze of lemon for flavour.
1 cup of black coffee or lemon tea

MID-MORNING
1 cup of lemon or herbal tea

LUNCH
Avocado salad made as follows:

Take ½ an avocado (you will have half left over from breakfast), remove the skin and cut into thin slices. Arrange on a plate with 1 hard boiled egg, also cut into thin slices, 4 halves of fresh peaches or apricots (if using tinned, be sure to drain off all the juice) plus a few slices of cucumber. Over the salad, squeeze the juice of 1 whole lemon.

Plus 1 cup of lemon or herbal tea

TEA-TIME
1 cup of tea with lemon

DINNER
3 oz. (75 g) of *one* of the following:

chicken, hot or cold, with the skin removed
beef
lamb
tuna fish, well drained
crab meat

Serve with 2 tablespoons cooked carrots (try to use fresh ones). Do not overcook them, but keep them quite firm, then drain and toss in the juice of 1 lemon and a little salt and black pepper and chopped parsley. Serve on a separate side plate.

For dessert, you have ½ an avocado cut into thin slices and served with a sauce made from ½ a small carton of natural yoghurt. To this you add 1 teaspoon runny honey. Mix together and pour over the avocado slices.

Plus 1 cup of lemon or herbal tea

Here are a couple of useful hints about avocados. If your avocado is hard when you buy it, wrap it in newspaper and leave in a warm room for a couple of days. Then, if you gently press the stalk end, it should be soft and ready to use.

To serve, always cut the avocado lengthwise, remove stone, and brush with lemon juice. This will prevent discoloration.

BOVRIL DIET
(average weight loss 4 lb. in two days)

Bovril as a meat extract is both nourishing and sustaining. The calorie value is very low – only approximately ten calories per cup. On the Bovril Diet you eat five times a day and, although the quantities are small, you will not feel hungry.

BREAKFAST
1 small glass of any natural fruit juice, unsweetened
1 small cup of black coffee
1 slice of low-calorie bread or crispbread, thinly spread with butter and a little Bovril

11 AM
1 cup of Bovril
2 tablespoons cottage cheese, sprinkled with Lee & Perrin sauce or soya sauce
Either a stick of celery to nibble with the cheese
Or 2 large tomato halves, spread thinly with mustard and grilled

2 PM
Either 3 tablespoons of any fresh fruit salad
Or 2 halves of grapefruit sprinkled with cheese and grilled
Or cucumber and mushroom salad made from ½ a chopped cucumber plus 5 chopped raw mushrooms, sprinkled with lemon juice

Plus 1 cup of Bovril

5 PM
Either 2 slices of lean bacon spread very thinly with Bovril and grilled. Eat with one thin slice of melon.
Or 1 boiled egg to be eaten with 1 thin crispbread spread with a little butter and Bovril
Or 1 thin crispbread spread with a little butter and Bovril and topped with 2 oz. (50 g) of hard cheese plus 2 gherkins

Plus 1 cup of tea or black coffee

8 PM
1 cup of Bovril
1 piece of any fresh fruit

DESPERATE DIET
(average weight loss 4–5 lb. in two days)

This marvellous diet consists of only three things – apple juice, cottage cheese and melon. Everyone I have given the diet to has never failed to lose weight – try it and see!

Breakfast, lunch and dinner on each of the two days are exactly the same:

1 glass of apple juice
4 oz. (125 g) carton of cottage cheese
2 medium slices of melon, served with a wedge of lemon

Eat and drink only what is in the diet and try to remember to weigh yourself each day.

ORANGE AND GRAPEFRUIT DIET
(average weight loss 3–4 lb. in two days)

This simple yet effective diet is rich in Vitamin C and, as well as aiding weight loss, it is an ideal health improvement diet for the whole family, since you could serve the salad as a dessert or as a summer breakfast dish to non-dieters. It is not an expensive diet and the fruit salad combination is quite delicious.

For one day's supply of the orange and grapefruit salad, you will need:

4 oranges, peeled and quartered
3 grapefruits, peeled and quartered
10–12 raisins
4 chopped dates
1 diced carrot
dressing of lemon, vinegar, honey and parsley

Method
Put all ingredients in a bowl and toss well together, then add a dressing made from 1 dessertspoon of lemon juice, 1 teaspoon of white wine vinegar, 2 teaspoons of honey and 2–3 sprigs of chopped parsley.

BREAKFAST
1 small glass of hot water, with ½ teaspoon honey stirred in
2 tablespoons orange and grapefruit salad
1 small cup of black coffee

MID-MORNING
the juice of 1 orange and 1 grapefruit mixed together with ½ teaspoon honey and 1 glass of hot water

LUNCH
2 tablespoons orange and grapefruit salad
1 cup of black coffee

TEA-TIME
1 cup of lemon tea
1 dry biscuit

DINNER
3 slices of any lean meat, hot or cold, but without gravy or sauce, served with 1 grilled tomato
3 tablespoons orange and grapefruit salad
1 cup of black coffee

LAST MINUTE DIET
(average weight loss 4–5 lb. in two days)

I designed this diet to give the maximum benefit from summer fresh fruits, high in vitamins and minerals and natural health-giving qualities. The ideal time to follow this diet is mid-summer when summer fruits are at their best.

BREAKFAST
Into a small glass dish place the following:

8–10 destalked strawberries, loganberries or raspberries
8–10 blackcurrants
8–10 cubes of fresh melon

Mix together and sprinkle with the juice of a fresh orange.

You may also have 1 glass of yoghurt health drink, which is made as follows:

Add a small carton of natural yoghurt to a glass filled with ice. Mix well and it is then ready to drink. If you like, a little honey can be added.

Plus 1 small black coffee, herbal tea or tea with lemon

LUNCH
A summer fruit plate, made as follows:

Wash and prepare 1 cup of *either* strawberries, raspberries *or* loganberries. Cut into slices 1 banana, a 3-inch wedge of watermelon and ¾ of a cucumber. Put all into a large glass bowl. Mix 1 teaspoon mint jelly with lemon juice and pour over the fruit. Arrange on a large plate, and finally sprinkle with 2 teaspoons of salted peanuts.

Plus 1 glass of yoghurt health drink as for breakfast

TEA-TIME
1 cup of herbal tea or tea with lemon

DINNER
Exactly the same as for breakfast

It would be a good idea to vary the fruit at meal-times. For example if you take strawberries for breakfast, then take loganberries for lunch, and vice versa.

PANIC STATIONS DIET
(average weight loss 5 lb. in two days)

Here is a wonderful quickie diet that doesn't involve too much effort. It is based on a healthful slimming drink which is taken three times a day in place of normal meals, together with a delicious fruit and nut dish.

At each meal-time, 3 times a day, mix together the following:

6 tablespoons apple juice
6 tablespoons orange juice
1½ teaspoons fresh lemon or lime juice
1 teaspoon fresh plain yoghurt
1 teaspoon condensed milk or runny honey

Method
Mix all ingredients together thoroughly and drink slowly in small sips as this aids the digestion better than one large gulp.

With the drink you may have a dish of *either* 10–12 fresh strawberries *or* 2 fresh pears, thinly sliced, *or* 2 fresh peaches, thinly sliced, *or* 1 large banana, peeled and sliced. To the fruit add *either* 10–12 walnuts *or* hazelnuts *or* almonds, and a squeeze of fresh lemon.

Plus in between meals you may have 1 cup of either mint or herbal tea, or tea without milk, but you should not exceed 3 cups per day

STRAWBERRY DIET
(average weight loss 5 lb. in two days)

Even if you are not a strawberry addict, I feel sure this diet will appeal to you, since it is so easy to prepare and delicious to taste. Half a cup of fresh strawberries contain more Vitamin C than one fresh orange and, for maximum health, should be eaten as fresh as possible.

BREAKFAST
1 small glass of milk (about ¼ pint/150 ml)
5–6 fresh strawberries
1 teaspoon honey
a few ice cubes

Method
First mash strawberries and honey together in a tall glass, then add ice cubes and milk. Stir and drink at once.

Plus if you are still thirsty, 1 small cup of herbal tea or tea with lemon

MID-MORNING
1 small cup of herbal tea or tea with lemon

LUNCH
½ a melon, any variety
6–8 strawberries
1 dessertspoon chopped almonds
2 tablespoons natural yoghurt
2 teaspoons fresh lemon juice
1 teaspoon finely chopped mint

Method
First, cube melon and place in a bowl. Then add chopped strawberries and almonds. Mix lemon juice, yoghurt and mint together, and pour over the salad. It is ready to eat at once.

Plus you may also have 1 cup of herbal tea or tea with lemon; or why not try iced tea? It is delicious with this salad. You make it in a tall glass, adding one teabag, hot water to half-way up the glass, then lots of ice cubes and a slice of lemon.

TEA-TIME
1 small cup of herbal tea or tea with lemon

DINNER
½ pint (275 ml) milk
5–6 fresh strawberries
1 teaspoon honey
a few ice cubes

Prepare strawberry cup as for breakfast, but note that the milk quantity is higher at dinner.

Plus 1 small cup of herbal tea or tea with lemon

Three-Day Diets

For best results these should be followed on three consecutive days. But if this is not possible you may diet on three alternating days in a week.

CHEESE AND TOMATO DIET
(average weight loss is 3 lb. in three days)

The new Cheese and Tomato Diet is an effective way of losing weight quickly without ever getting real hunger pangs. The diet can be followed quite painlessly for three days.

I suggest that when you try the diet you alternate it with a sensible eating plan consisting of plenty of grilled meats and fish, fresh vegetables and fruit.

BREAKFAST
1 small glass of tomato juice mixed together with the juice from ½ a lemon
3 oz. (75 g) Cheddar cheese, thinly sliced
2 crispbreads, each with a smear of margarine
1 thinly sliced tomato with a squeeze of lemon juice
cayenne pepper

Method
Arrange the cheese and tomato slices in alternate layers on the crispbreads. Top with a little cayenne pepper and a squeeze of lemon juice, and it is then ready to eat.

Plus 1 glass of tea with lemon, no sugar, but you may use an artificial sweetener

LUNCH
Hot cheese bake which is made from the following:

1 hard boiled egg
3 oz. (75 g) grated Cheddar cheese
2 tomatoes
1 eating apple
4–5 button mushrooms
the juice of 1 lemon
a pinch of curry powder

Method
Chop the egg, tomatoes, apple and mushrooms into small chunks and arrange in a small, shallow, slightly oiled dish. Then sprinkle on the curry powder and the lemon juice and cheese, and place under a hot grill until the cheese is hot and toasted.

Plus 1 glass of tea with lemon, no sugar, but you may use an artificial sweetener

DINNER
Tomato cocktail which is made as follows:

Put into a liquidiser 1 large glass of tomato juice, 1 carton of natural yoghurt, the juice of ½ a lemon, 1 teaspoon of Worcestershire sauce and 2 teaspoons of sherry. Blend all the ingredients together and serve in a tall glass.

Plus 1 finger size of Cheddar cheese to nibble on and 2 sticks of celery
1 glass of hot tea with lemon, no sugar, but you may use an artificial sweetener

MELON DIET
(average weight loss 5 lb. in three days)

This is an eight-meal-a-day diet, designed to ward off hunger pangs and really aid weight loss. Melons are an ideal slimmers' choice since, apart from their very low calorie value, they are delicious to eat and easily digestible.

Meal 1
8 AM
1 slice of melon sprinkled with the juice of a wedge of lemon
1 black coffee

Meal 2
10 AM
1 boiled egg with a little sea salt
1 cup of black coffee

Meal 3
12 NOON
1 slice of melon, sprinkled with the juice of a wedge of lemon
1 cup of black coffee

Meal 4
2 PM
1 oz. (25 g) blue cheese or Cheddar cheese, eaten with ½ a slice of melon. Cut cheese and melon into wedges and eat together.
1 small glass of cider or apple juice

Meal 5
4 PM
4–6 thickish slices of cucumber, including the skin. Cut into chunks and sprinkle with a little sea salt or a dash of soya sauce. Halve and add to this the melon slice left over from your 2 p.m. meal. Also add 1 stick of celery, if you have it, or a little watercress. Dress with fresh lemon juice and your salad is ready to eat.

Plus 1 cup of black coffee

Meal 6
6 PM
1 slice of melon

Meal 7
8 PM
1 slice of melon
2 lean slices of any cold meats
1 small glass of cider or apple juice

Meal 8
10 PM
1 smallish glass of hot milk
1 crispbread

The meals may be switched around, providing you do not add or change anything listed, but the hot milk should be your last meal of the day. Also, the black coffee permitted throughout the day should be small cups, such as after dinner coffee cups.

To make 1 melon last the whole day, cut in half, then cut each half in three and keep as cool as possible before serving.

NEW YEAR DIET
(average weight loss 5½ lb. in three days)

This diet is simple and effective and really does get results. It is ideal as an aid to quick weight loss after overindulgence at Christmas, when weight gain seems inevitable.

Day 1
BREAKFAST
½ a grapefruit
½ a banana
1 small carton of natural yoghurt
1 black coffee or tea with lemon

LUNCH
½ a grapefruit
½ a banana
1 boiled egg
1 black coffee or tea with lemon

DINNER
½ a grapefruit
½ a banana
1 small carton of cottage cheese
1 black coffee or tea with lemon

Day 2
BREAKFAST
½ a grapefruit
½ a banana
2 slices of very crispy grilled bacon
1 black coffee or tea with lemon

LUNCH
½ a grapefruit
½ a banana
4 thin slices of cold chicken *or* turkey
1 black coffee or tea with lemon

DINNER
½ a grapefruit
½ a banana
4 oz. (125 g) peeled shrimps with lemon
1 black coffee or tea with lemon

Day 3
BREAKFAST
½ a grapefruit
½ a banana
¼ pint (150 ml) glass of milk
1 black coffee or tea with lemon

LUNCH
½ a grapefruit
½ a banana
¼ pint (150 ml) glass of milk
1 black coffee or tea with lemon

DINNER
½ a grapefruit
½ a banana
¼ pint (150 ml) glass of milk
1 black coffee or tea with lemon

Sugar should not be added to either the grapefruit or the drink, but you may use an artificial sweetener.

QUICKIE FRUIT DIET
(average weight loss 6 lb. in three days)

Whatever your reasons are for leaving your diet to the last moment, don't despair, for the Quickie Fruit Diet really does work! The evening meal is delicious enough to eat as a starter or dessert even when you are not dieting.

BREAKFAST
½ a melon, whichever variety you like to choose, and eat with 1 apple, cut into quarters and spread with a little honey
1 glass of fruit juice
1 small cup of tea with lemon only

MID-MORNING
1 tangerine, orange or satsuma

LUNCH
1 large glass of fresh, tinned or frozen orange juice, to which you add 1 thinly sliced, mashed banana. Mix together and it is then ready to drink.

TEA-TIME
1 tangerine, orange or satsuma

DINNER
Take 1 whole grapefruit, cut in half and remove segments. Chop segments up together with 4–5 black or white grapes and 2 teaspoons of chopped almonds. Return mixture to shells, spread each with a teaspoon of runny honey and place under a hot grill for about 3–4 minutes.

Plus 1 cup of tea with lemon only

SUMMER DIET
(average weight loss 4 lb. in three days)

This diet can be followed for any three days in a week with an average weight loss of four pounds in three days, without ever feeling really hungry.

BREAKFAST
1 glass of lemon, herbal, or mint tea
1 fresh orange, peeled and served with a squeeze of lemon
1 finger-size wedge of hard cheese, to be eaten with the orange

MID-MORNING
1 glass of lemon, mint or herbal tea
1 fresh orange

LUNCH
A crunchy summer salad made from:

2 oranges
3 oz. (75 g) hard cheese
½ a cucumber
2 or 3 raw mushrooms
1 dessertspoon raisins
1 dessertspoon peanuts
the juice of 1 lemon
1½ teaspoons oil

Method
Peel and chop up the orange, cucumber and mushrooms, including the stalks. (If they are the small button ones, you do not have to peel them, just wash them.) Cube the cheese and mix together. Combine the oil and lemon and pour over the salad, and then finally toss in the raisins and peanuts.

Plus 1 glass of lemon, mint or herbal tea

TEA-TIME
1 glass of lemon, mint or herbal tea
1 fresh orange

DINNER
Mix and eat together 1 fresh orange, segmented, 1 tablespoon raisins and 1 tablespoon peanuts.

Plus 1 glass of lemon, mint or herbal tea

TANTALISING DIET
(average weight loss 5 lb. in three days)

A three-day diet designed to help you lose weight, which at the same time allows you to eat tantalising foods in moderation without the fear of gaining pounds.

BREAKFAST
1 boiled egg, with salt and pepper
1 small brown roll with a smear of margarine
1 cup of jasmine tea

LUNCH
½ an avocado, dressed with lemon juice
4 oz. (125 g) plain cottage cheese, which you could pile into your avocado pear, then sprinkle with freshly chopped chives and parsley
A long cool drink made by mixing 1 glass of Pouilly Fuissé (white wine) with 1 glass of bottled water, ice cubes and a slice of lemon

DINNER
Either up to ½ hot or cold small roast chicken, no skin. Serve on a bed of fresh watercress and with a wedge of lemon.
Or ½ a lobster, grilled without sauce or butter, but served with a watercress salad topped with thin onion rings and dressed with a teaspoon of oil and a wedge of lemon.

Plus 1 long cool drink, as for lunch and 1 small black coffee, if you really need it

If you are really thirsty during the day, you may have up to three average-sized glasses of bottled mineral water only.

SIMPLE BANANA DIET
(average weight loss 4lb. in three days)

This Banana Diet could not be easier since, except for the evening meal, no cooking is involved. The results are very good – one client of mine lost six pounds in three days with this diet and, although a busy working girl, did not feel any hunger pangs.

BREAKFAST
1 banana
1 glass of skimmed milk or non-fat powdered milk
1 small cup of black coffee

MID-MORNING
1 small cup of black coffee

LUNCH
1 banana
3 tablespoons cottage cheese or 3 oz. (75 g) hard cheese
1 cup of black coffee

TEA-TIME
1 cup of tea with lemon

DINNER
4–6 oz. (125–175 g) steak, grilled, served with watercress
1 banana, which could be peeled, cut lengthwise, and grilled with the steak. Or simply eat it cold as a dessert after the steak.
1 cup of black coffee or tea with lemon

Four-Day Diets

Like the three-day diets, these can either be followed on consecutive days for really good results or on a two day on/two day off basis. An easy to follow routine would be four days out of every eight over a two-week period. This should be very rewarding and also not too boring.

APPLE AND CHEESE DIET
(average weight loss 5 lb. in four days)

This diet is made up of two main ingredients, apple and cheese, a really delicious combination. It is very simple to prepare, tasty and not expensive.

BREAKFAST
Either 1 large raw eating apple, peeled and cut into thin slices. Spread on a plate and sprinkle with a little lemon juice and cinnamon.
Or 2 medium cooking apples, stewed with a little cinnamon and lemon juice. Eat either hot or cold.
Or if you are in a hurry, just nibble one large eating apple, the skin as well.

Plus 2 oz. (50 g) of hard cheese
1 cup of coffee or tea with milk; no sugar but you may use an artificial sweetener

MID-MORNING
Welsh rarebit made with 1 oz. (25 g) of grated cheese and 1 slice of slimming bread. You may use a little margarine on the bread.
Either 1 medium glass of apple juice *or* cider *or* tea with lemon

LUNCH
You may have one of the breakfast dishes and the cheese
Either 1 medium glass of apple juice *or* cider *or* tea with lemon

TEA-TIME
Either 1 cup of tea with milk or lemon *or* 1 medium glass of apple juice

DINNER
Apple and cheese burger, made as follows:

Peel and core 1 very large cooking apple, and cut into 4 thick round slices. Then spread each slice with a smear of honey, and grill till lightly browned. Turn and grill on the other side, but be sure not to overcook the apple. Then remove from the grill and sprinkle each slice with approximately 2 teaspoons of finely grated cheese. Place under the grill again for about 1 minute or until the cheese has melted. Then serve on a bed of lettuce with 3 or 4 thin raw onion rings.

Plus either 1 medium glass of apple juice *or* cider *or* tea with lemon

AYRAM HEALTH DIET
(average weight loss 5 lb. in four days)

This is a Turkish diet, designed to rid the body of toxins and to give the digestive organs a periodic rest. Ayram is a Turkish word for a health-giving drink made from natural yoghurt and water. The diet also includes lapa (plain boiled rice). As the first day is only liquids, I suggest you rest as much as possible.

Day 1
8 AM
1 glass of ayram made as follows:

Fill a ¼ pint (150 ml) glass with natural yoghurt and mix well with ¼ pint (150 ml) of cold mineral water. It is then ready to drink.

2 PM
1 glass of ayram

4 PM
1 glass of ayram

8 PM
1 glass of ayram

In addition to the ayram, throughout the day you may have up to 5 cups of *either* black coffee or tea without milk or sugar. *Or* you may have the same quantity of mineral water.

Day 2
8 AM
1 plate of approximately 3 tablespoons lapa (plain boiled rice without salt)
1 glass of ayram

10 AM
1 glass of ayram

12 NOON
1 plate of 3 tablespoons lapa
1 glass of ayram

4 PM
1 glass of ayram

6 PM
1 plate of 3 tablespoons lapa
1 glass of ayram

8 PM
1 glass of ayram

In addition to the ayram and lapa, throughout the day you may have up to 3 cups of *either* black coffee or tea without milk and sugar. *Or* you may have the same quantity of mineral water.

Day 3
The same as Day 1

Day 4
The same as Day 2

The additional drinks should only be taken if you really need them.

CHEESE DIET
(average weight loss 6 lb. in four days)

Cheese is a wonderful way of taking in protein and keeping the calories down at the same time. The kind of cheese you eat on a slimming diet is most important as it can vary from 98 calories per ounce (25 g) to 300 calories. The least fattening and the most sustaining, are Edam, Gouda and Cheddar.

ON RISING
The juice of 1 whole lemon, drunk naturally on its own

BREAKFAST
1 cup of tea or coffee, with a little milk but no sugar
1 piece of any fresh fruit of your choice
2 starch-reduced crispbreads, spread with a little butter and topped with a little slice of Edam, Gouda or Cheddar cheese

MID-MORNING
1 glass of lemonade made from fresh lemons only, with ½ teaspoon honey to sweeten

LUNCH
A minty platter made with:

1 good slice of Edam chese
1 good slice of Gouda cheese
1 hard boiled egg
1 apple
1 orange
a few grapes
½ a banana
dressing of mint jelly, orange and vinegar

Method
Arrange all the ingredients on a large plate and serve with a mint dressing made the following way: take 2 teaspoons of mint jelly, plus the juice of ½ an orange and a dash of vinegar. Mix all well together and pour over the platter.

Plus 1 fresh yoghurt
1 cup of tea or coffee, with a little milk but no sugar

TEA-TIME
1 glass of fresh lemonade as before

DINNER
Exactly the same as for breakfast

HONEY, MILK AND ALMOND DIET
(average weight loss 5 lb. in four days)

Most of the ingredients for this diet you will probably already have in your kitchen, so no special shopping is required. The diet is simple to prepare, sustaining and delicious to taste.

ON RISING
1 cup of tea with milk, but no sugar

BREAKFAST
Heat ½ pint (275 ml) of milk slowly in a saucepan, and add 1 dessertspoon ground almonds and 1 dessertspoon runny honey. Then slowly add a beaten egg. Stir gradually. Do not let the mixture boil and then when hot, serve in a mug with a pinch of grated nutmeg on top.

Plus 1 piece of fresh fruit of your choice

LUNCH
A honey almond salad made from the following:

1 × 4 oz. (125 g) carton of cottage cheese
½ a cup of yoghurt
1 dessertspoon runny honey
1 dessertspoon coarsely chopped almonds
1 dessertspoon raisins and sultanas
1 peeled and chopped apple *or* pear *or* 3 plums
lettuce

Method
Mix together cottage cheese, honey and yoghurt in a bowl. Then fold in the nuts, raisins and sultanas, apple *or* pear *or* plums, and serve on a bed of crisp lettuce.

Plus 1 cup of tea or coffee with milk, but no sugar

DINNER
Exactly the same as for breakfast, but omit the egg and add 1 dessertspoon of brandy, if you wish

Try not to drink between meals.

LIBERAL DIET
(average weight loss 4 lb. in four days)

This is a more liberal eating plan of the World's Cheapest Diet in the One-Day Diets section of this book, which includes the potato water because it is so good for the health and skin.

BREAKFAST
1 small glass of potato water (see One-Day Diets section for recipe)
3 grilled tomatoes
½ a slice of toasted bread *or* 1 starch-reduced crispbread, with a little margarine
1 cup of tea with lemon

MID-MORNING
1 small glass of potato water

LUNCH
1 small bowl of any clear soup
2 starch-reduced crispbreads, spread with 2 oz. (50 g) of cottage cheese and topped with a few slices of pickled gherkin
1 cup of tea with lemon

TEA-TIME
1 small glass of potato water

DINNER
Take 2 of your already parboiled potatoes (medium size). Peel and cut them into paper-thin slices. Then place a thin layer on the bottom of a well-greased, ovenproof dish and sprinkle with salt, pepper and a little grated cheese. Continue with the next layer, and so on, finishing with a layer of grated cheese (you will need about 2 oz. (50 g) of cheese altogether). Add 1 or 2 dots of margarine and bake in a moderate oven for 15–20 minutes.

Plus either 1 poached egg *or* 3 oz. (75 g) of grilled or plain baked white fish or grilled meat
1 cup of tea with lemon

BEFORE RETIRING
1 small glass of potato water

ORANGE COCKTAIL AND CHEESE DIET
(average weight loss 5 lb. in four days)

This diet has been one of the most successful I have ever designed. Men and women all over the country who tried it had the most amazing results. The diet is so simple: cheese and oranges, a wonderful combination. Refreshing and delicious to eat.

Make one day's supply of the orange cocktail as follows:

Take 6 medium-sized oranges, peel, quarter and cut segments in half. Over these, squeeze out the juice of 2 lemons, and add 3 tablespoons of concentrated orange squash. This will give the fruit a delicious sort of liqueur flavour. Toss the segments well into the juice, and keep cold in the refrigerator until you are ready to eat.

BREAKFAST
1 portion of orange cocktail
1 black coffee or tea with lemon, but no sugar

MID-MORNING
1 tumbler of mineral water

LUNCH
1 portion of orange cocktail
3 oz. (75 g) Cheddar cheese
1 black coffee or tea with lemon, but no sugar

TEA-TIME
1 cup of tea with lemon but no sugar

DINNER
Either a 2-egg-omelette with 1 oz. (25 g) grated cheese
Or 2 baked eggs, topped with 1 oz. (25 g) of grated cheese
Or 2 hard boiled eggs with 1 oz. (25 g) of cheese to nibble on

Plus 1 portion of orange cocktail
1 glass of either dry white wine or sherry
1 small black coffee, if you need it

BEFORE RETIRING
1 glass of mineral water

The orange cocktail is delicious enough to eat even when you are not on a diet and is an ideal dessert to serve after a very heavy main course.

WINTER VITAMIN CUP DIET
(average weight loss 5 lb. in four days)

This diet is ideal for those people who have little or no time to eat proper meals but are in need of stamina and energy. If you are a working person, then you can prepare it beforehand and take it in a flask with you. But shake well before drinking.

The vitamin cup is taken for breakfast and lunch, in place of your normal meals, and you may have as much black coffee or lemon tea as you want, but no sugar. Use an artificial sweetener if necessary.

For one meal's supply of the vitamin cup:

½ pint (275 ml) of tomato juice
2 tablespoons plain yoghurt
1 teaspoon Yeastamin
1 raw egg
2 tablespoons milk

Method
Blend all the ingredients well together, and it is then ready to drink. If you do not have an electric blender or liquidiser, first beat the egg well until it is frothy, then mix in the Yeastamin and gradually add all the other ingredients, and whisk for a few minutes.

DINNER
Up to 6 oz. (175 g) of meat, cooked any way except in a rich sauce or pie-crust
2 green vegetables *or* 1 large green mixed salad. With the salad you may have a little French dressing, but no mayonnaise.
1 glass of either dry white wine *or* sherry *or* soda water
1 small black coffee or tea with lemon

One-Week Diets

A whole week of dieting does take some effort and determination, but if you have a particular goal in mind or a special occasion at which you want to look your best then the effort is worth it. Usually, as with all diets, the first two days are the most difficult, but once you have dieted for a whole week and lost some weight, the incentive to continue and maintain those results grows stronger.

EASY DIET
(average weight loss is 4 lb. in one week)

Day 1
BREAKFAST
1 whole orange
1 boiled egg
1 crispbread, spread with margarine
1 small coffee or tea with milk only

LUNCH
1 small carton of cottage cheese
1 tomato
¼ cucumber
1 small coffee or tea, with milk only, or 1 glass of mineral water

DINNER
1 small bowl of clear bouillon soup
2 lean, grilled lamb cutlets, with mint sauce
1 tablespoon boiled carrots
1 tablespoon courgettes
1 apple
1 small coffee or tea, with milk only or 1 glass of mineral water

Day 2
BREAKFAST
6–8 stewed prunes
1 thin slice of toasted wholemeal bread with a covering of a thin slice of Edam, Gouda or Cheddar cheese
1 small coffee or tea, with milk only

LUNCH
1 tablespoon well drained tuna fish served with lemon and watercress, and chopped raw mushrooms
1 small tea or coffee, with milk only or 1 glass of mineral water

DINNER
½ a grapefruit, without sugar
3 thin slices of sautéd liver
1 small potato
1 tablespoon French or runner beans
1 fruit yoghurt
1 small coffee or tea, with milk only or 1 glass of mineral water

Day 3
BREAKFAST
4–6 stewed apricots
1 egg, scrambled
1 crispbread, spread with margarine
1 small coffee or tea, with milk only

LUNCH
2 thin slices of ham, corned beef, or tongue
2 slices of fresh or tinned pineapple
1 tablespoon coleslaw
1 small coffee or tea, with milk only or 1 glass of mineral water

DINNER
1 large slice of melon
4–6 oz. (125–175 g) chicken, without the skin
2 tablespoons spinach, with lemon
2 tablespoons fresh fruit salad
1 small coffee or tea, with milk only or 1 glass of mineral water

Day 4
BREAKFAST
4–6 stewed figs
1 crispbread spread with margarine and a little marmalade or honey
1 cup of coffee or tea, with milk only

LUNCH
2-egg omelette, filled with mushrooms
1 small coffee or tea, with milk only or 1 glass of mineral water

DINNER
1 tablespoon peeled shrimps, with lemon
a very thin slice of brown wholemeal bread spread with margarine
an average portion of casserole, with a small green salad and a little French dressing
1 fresh pear
1 small coffee or tea, with milk only or 1 glass of mineral water

Day 5
BREAKFAST
2 tablespoons stewed, unsweetened apple
1 poached egg, with a crispbread and margarine
1 small coffee or tea, with milk only

LUNCH
1 cup of Bovril or Marmite
2 large slices of Edam, Gouda or Cheddar cheese
1 apple
2 sticks of celery
1 small coffee or tea, with milk only or 1 glass of mineral water

DINNER
½ a grapefruit, without sugar
3 slices of roast lamb, with pickled cucumber
1 tablespoon peas
1 tablespoon sprouts or cabbage
1 small creme caramel
1 small coffee or tea, with milk only or 1 glass of mineral water

Day 6
BREAKFAST
1 small bowl of cereal with milk, no sugar
1 crispbread, with a thin slice of Edam, Cheddar or Gouda cheese
1 small coffee or tea, with milk only

LUNCH
1 chopped, hard boiled egg served on a bed of chopped lettuce, red and green peppers and fresh onion, with a little French dressing
1 small coffee or tea, with milk only or 1 glass of mineral water

DINNER
1 small bowl of clear bouillon soup
an average portion of grilled, baked or steamed white fish, served with a wedge of lemon
1 tablespoon green beans
1 tablespoon sautéd mushrooms
1 orange
1 small coffee or tea, with milk only or 1 glass of mineral water

Day 7
BREAKFAST
1 fresh peach
1 carton of natural yoghurt with bran
1 small coffee or tea, with milk only

LUNCH
1 grilled hamburger, without bun
1 tablespoon chips *or* 1 small jacket potato
1 small coffee or tea, with milk only or 1 glass of mineral water

DINNER
½ a grapefruit, grilled and served hot
1 poached egg, served on a bed of lighty buttered spinach
1 tablespoon fruit jelly or ice-cream
1 small coffee or tea, with milk only or 1 glass of mineral water

EIGHT MEALS A DAY DIET
(average weight loss 6 lb. in one week)

One of the most difficult tasks for slimmers to overcome is nibbling between meals. With this in mind, I planned the Eight Meals a Day Diet and I feel it is the answer to compulsive nibblers' weight loss regime.

7.30 AM
1 small glass of grapefruit juice, preferably unsweetened
Either ½ a grapefruit *or* a small slice of melon

9 AM
1 small cup of coffee with milk only
Either 1 lightly boiled egg with a little salt *or* 1 thin slice of brown or wholemeal bread spread with a little margarine *or* 1 glass of milk with a raw egg beaten into it and a pinch of nutmeg (if you choose this, do not have the coffee)

11.30 AM
Either 1 apple, orange or pear
Or 1 tablespoon cottage cheese and 2 finely chopped dates, mixed together

1 PM
You may choose *one* of the following dishes:

(i) 1 small bowl of any clear soup, or soup made with a bouillon cube. You may also have a finger of cheese cut into small pieces which you add to the soup.

(ii) 1 tablespoon of really well drained tuna fish or salmon. With this you could eat a good portion of mustard and cress, or watercress, or chopped raw cabbage, dressed with a little lemon juice only.

Plus 1 cup of lemon tea without sugar

3.30 PM
Either the other half of the grapefruit left over from breakfast, served as before, or you could grill it and eat it hot
Or 1 natural yoghurt

5 PM
1 dry starch-reduced biscuit
1 small cup of lemon tea or black coffee

7.30 PM
2 slices of any meat, hot or cold, without fat
1 small potato, boiled *or* 1 grilled tomato
3 grilled mushrooms, medium size
1 poached egg
1 small glass of any fruit juice or mineral water

9 PM
1 small glass of your usual nightcap, but without sugar if it is a sweet drink
1 dry starch-reduced crispbread

FINAL DIET
(average weight loss 5 lb. in one week)

This diet, regardless of age, really does show good results in a week, providing you are strong-willed enough not to cheat or substitute foods other than those specified.

BREAKFAST
1 medium glass of any unsweetened fruit juice, preferably fresh
Either 1 slice of melon
Or ½ a grapefruit, with the juice of ½ an orange squeezed on it
Or 1 lightly boiled egg

Plus 1 small black coffee or tea with lemon, no sugar

MID-MORNING
If you are very thirsty, you may have a wine glass of pure lemon juice, without sugar, but an artificial sweetener is allowed

LUNCH
You may have one of the following dishes:

(i) 4 oz. (125 g) of low fat cottage cheese with 2 tablespoons of fresh fruit salad, no juice

(ii) 2 starch-reduced crispbreads. On these you can have 1 oz. (25 g) of any cheese, except cream cheese plus as many slices of cucumber and tomato as you want.

(iii) 1 hard boiled egg, if you did not have one for breakfast, and a salad of 1 tomato, cucumber and lettuce and some grated fresh onion with a little French dressing

Plus 1 cup of black coffee or tea with lemon, without sugar, but you can use an artificial sweetener

TEA-TIME
The same drink as for mid-morning

DINNER
You may choose *one* of the following:

(i) 4 oz. (125 g) of either steamed or grilled sole, plaice, fresh haddock, or cod. If grilling, use a little oil.

(ii) 4 oz. (125 g) of lean cooked veal, chicken or liver, grilled only

(iii) 2 eggs, boiled, poached, or baked, but do not choose eggs if taken at breakfast or lunch

To accompany the above, you may have *either* 4 large tablespoons of any 2 of the following vegetables: broccoli, Brussels sprouts, cauliflower, runner beans, leeks, grilled tomato *or* a large mixed green salad

Do not have sauces, gravy or salad cream with your dinner, and keep the salt to a minimum. But as a dressing on the vegetables, you can have lemon juice, and 1 dessertspoon of dressing on the salad made from vinegar or lemon.

Plus 1 of the following fruits as a dessert: apple, peach, pear, orange, up to 4 oz. (125 g) of cherries, fresh strawberries or grapes, without cream or sugar. Make sure the fruit is fresh.

1 cup of black coffee or lemon tea

No wine or alcohol – save this for your holiday!

FRUIT AND VEGETABLE ALTERNATING DIET
(average weight loss 8 lb. in one week)

This fruit and vegetable diet is an ideal way of giving the tummy a rest and at the same time helps to build up in the body the vitamin and mineral content so often lacking in the bland diets of today.

The Fruit Day
BREAKFAST
1 glass of any fresh fruit juice
2 tomatoes and 2 fresh pineapple slices
Sprinkle both with cinnamon, and place under a hot grill for about 5 minutes. Serve with a wedge of lemon.

Plus 1 cup of herbal, mint or lemon tea

LUNCH
Fresh fruit salad, made from:
1 apple
1 pear
6 grapes
2 dates
1 fresh slice of pineapple
1 orange
dressing of cinnamon, paprika and lemon

Method
Peel and finely chop up all the salad ingredients and place in a dish. Sprinkle with cinnamon and paprika, and the juice of 1 lemon.

Plus 1 cup of herbal, mint or lemon tea

DINNER
1 very large banana, or 2 small bananas, peeled and cut lengthwise. Spread with a little honey, cinnamon and lemon juice, and place under a hot grill for about 5 minutes. Serve on a bed of ice cold melon chunks.

Plus 1 cup of herbal, mint or lemon tea

BEFORE RETIRING
1 tumbler of warm water

The Vegetable Day
BREAKFAST
1 glass of any fresh vegetable juice

6 large, or 12 small, button mushrooms and 3 small courgettes served as follows: Peel and cut the vegetables lengthwise. Sprinkle with a little salt and lemon juice, and grill for about 10 minutes. Serve hot.

Plus 1 cup of herbal, mint or lemon tea

LUNCH
Made from the following:

2 sticks of celery, plus their tops
2 tablespoons cooked, but cold, French beans
1 small beetroot
1 small fresh leek, raw
1 small cold, cooked potato
dressing of oil, vinegar, mustard, salt and mixed herbs

Method
Chop up all the salad ingredients, place in a bowl and toss in a dressing made with 1 teaspoon of oil, 1 teaspoon of vinegar, ½ teaspoon of fresh or American mustard and garlic salt with a pinch of mixed herbs.

Plus 1 cup of herbal, mint or lemon tea

DINNER
1 bowl of spring or mixed vegetable soup
A vegetable salad made with 1 tablespoon cooked fresh carrots, 1 tablespoon cooked fresh peas, 1 small raw onion, finely chopped, 3–4 fresh asparagus spears, cooked. Serve the vegetables with a good knob of margarine and a wedge of lemon, salt and pepper to taste. Sprinkle chopped raw onion on top.

Plus 1 cup of herbal, mint or lemon tea

BEFORE RETIRING
1 tumbler of warm water

FRUITS OF SUMMER DIET
(average weight loss 6 lb. in one week)

The importance of eating raw foods cannot be stressed enough. They provide the essential vitamins and minerals for good health. Always cut and prepare only what you need for each meal and eat immediately. This particular diet gives maximum freshness and nutritive build-up.

ON RISING
1 glass of herbal tea

BREAKFAST
A salad, made from:

1 bowl of fresh strawberries
1 cup of natural yoghurt
1 teaspoon finely-chopped, fresh mint leaves
1 heaped tablespoon milled nuts

Method
Halve the strawberries, sprinkle over the milled nuts, pour on the yoghurt and finally add the chopped mint.

Plus 1 cup of herbal or China tea

MID-MORNING
1 glass of freshly-squeezed orange and lemon juice, mixed together

LUNCH
A salad made with strawberries, raspberries, currants (red, black or white), carrots, finely grated onions, young raw green peas, fresh spinach leaves, and fine herbs such as basil, dill, parsley. Dress salad with oil, lemon and black pepper only.

Plus 1 glass of herbal tea served with ice-cubes and a few sprigs of fresh mint

TEA-TIME
1 cup of herbal tea

DINNER
1 two-egg omelette *or* 2 oz. (50 g) cheese or tuna fish, served with a salad of lettuce and sorrel leaves, beetroot, celery, and finely grated cauliflower. Add a dressing of fresh orange juice, lemon juice, oil and natural yoghurt and crushed almonds.

Plus 1 glass of freshly squeezed orange and lemon juice mixed together

BEFORE RETIRING
1 cup of herbal or mint tea, to aid relaxation

GOURMET DIET
(average weight loss 4½ lb. in one week)

No one should complain about dieting on this diet, since the variation and choice is very wide, with delicious recipes and a glass of wine included every day. (Recipes marked with an asterisk are given in full below.)

Day 1
BREAKFAST (the same every day)
1 fresh orange or ½ a grapefruit
Either 1 egg, boiled, poached, baked or scrambled
Or 1 rasher of grilled, lean bacon with mushroom and tomato
Or a grilled kipper or poached smoked haddock

LUNCH
Grilled trout meunière with broccoli
orange and apricot mousse*

DINNER
Fresh asparagus with ¼ oz. (7½ g) of melted butter
baked veal savoyard* with French beans and courgettes, boiled
wild strawberries, with a little lemon juice and no sugar
1 glass of white wine

Day 2
LUNCH
Steak tartare with a cucumber and onion salad, flavoured with fresh dill
1 slice of fresh pineapple

DINNER
Artichoke hearts with lemon dressing*
grilled chicken rubbed with lemon and tarragon
spinach, served with grilled tomatoes
1 crispbread with 1 oz. (25 g) of Edam cheese, and a little watercress
1 glass of wine

One-Week Diets 57

Day 3
LUNCH
Stuffed tomatoes* with a green salad of cos lettuce and spring onion and a little lemon dressing
Either 1 fresh orange
Or 1 crispbread with 1 oz. (25 g) of Edam cheese

DINNER
Lemon soup*
cold lobster with avocado and chicory salad and a little vinaigrette dressing
fresh raspberries and a little cream
1 glass of wine

Day 4
LUNCH
Smoked salmon with 1 thin slice of wholemeal bread and a little butter and a squeeze of lemon
Either 1 fresh peach
Or 1 orange

DINNER
Prawns with 1 thin slice of wholemeal bread and a little butter
a lamb chop, flavoured with rosemary, and served with runner beans and 1 small potato, boiled in its jacket
1 fresh pear
1 oz. (25 g) of Edam cheese
1 glass of wine

Day 5
LUNCH
Spanish omelette and green salad with fresh mint and parsley
a compote of fresh cherries, grapes, plums and prunes

DINNER
Consommé
fresh salmon and cucumber salad
bilberry flan with a thin base of pastry and a little cream
1 glass of wine

Day 6
LUNCH
Iced tomato juice
a grilled fillet steak rubbed with garlic, served with a mixed green salad
sliced fresh peaches and oranges, sprinkled with 5 whole cloves, and decorated with mint leaves

DINNER
Gaspacho soup
red mullet, grilled, with cauliflower and a watercress and chicory salad
rhubarb fool, made with yoghurt not cream
1 glass of wine

Day 7
LUNCH
Roast guinea fowl with French beans and carrots
wild blackberry crumble (a thin topping of crumble only) and a little cream

DINNER
Cold meat served with either a tomato salad with lemon dressing, flavoured with basil and watercress or salad niçoise

Plus either 1 fresh orange *or* 1 thin crispbread
1 oz. (25 g) of Edam cheese
2 radishes
1 glass of wine

Here are the recipes for the dishes marked with an asterisk in the Gourmet Diet:

Orange and Apricot Mousse (serves 6–8)
1 large tin of apricots
3 oranges, washed and sliced with their peel on
3–4 whole cloves
½ pint (275 ml) natural yoghurt
a little grated nutmeg

Method
Tip apricots and oranges into a saucepan and bring to the

boil, stirring occasionally. Add cloves and nutmeg. Cover and simmer for 20 minutes. Allow to cool a little, then place in a blender. Once the mixture is smooth, remove and place on one side until it is cold. Stir in yoghurt, mix thoroughly, and then place in individual dishes and chill overnight before serving.

Baked Veal Savoyard (serves 4)
4 escalopes of veal
4 slices of lean ham
4 large slices of Edam cheese
seasoning
a little butter

Method
Season the escalopes, and wrap each one in a slice of ham. Place the wrapped escalopes in an ovenproof dish, and top each with a slice of Edam cheese. Dot with butter and cook for 1½ hours on Gas Mark 6, or 400°F/200°C.

Lemon Dressing (for the artichoke hearts) (serves 6)
freshly squeezed lemon juice from 3 lemons
salt
freshly ground black pepper
½ clove of garlic or garlic salt
2 teaspoons chopped fresh mint or dried mint
2 tablespoons soured cream or natural yoghurt

Method
Place all ingredients in a bowl, and blend together thoroughly.

Stuffed Tomatoes (serves 4)
8 medium-sized tomatoes
½ lb. (225 g) Edam cheese, grated
2 teaspoons chopped chives
2 teaspoons chopped fresh basil
2 oz. (50 g) chopped ham
salt
pepper
paprika
2 oz. (50 g) olives

Method
Wash tomatoes, remove stalks and cut wide slices off the top of each. Scoop out the inside of each with a teaspoon, taking care not to break the skin. Mix the cheese, chopped ham and herbs, and season with pepper, salt and a pinch of paprika. Fill the hollow tomato shells with the mixture, and decorate with black olives. Serve chilled on a bed of watercress.

Lemon Soup (serves 4)
1 egg
1 chicken stock cube
1 pint water
juice and grated peel of 1 lemon
1 medium-sized onion
5 cloves
1 oz. (25 g) Edam cheese
salt
freshly ground black pepper
a little fresh chopped parsley

Method
Peel onion and stick the cloves into it. Dissolve chicken stock in 1 pint (575 ml) boiling water and add onion. Continue boiling in a covered pan for 5 minutes, then reduce heat and simmer until onion is tender. Add lemon juice and grated peel, salt and black pepper. Immediately before serving, drop in the egg and stir until the soup is creamy. Garnish with grated cheese and fresh parsley.

SUPER DIET
(average weight loss 5 lb. in one week)

I have given the one-week Super Diet to many of my clients with amazing results. The secret of this diet is its simplicity, and no special shopping is required. Remember, no cheating and no substitutes will make the diet really effective.

BREAKFAST
1 small cup of black coffee, no sugar
1 fresh orange, eaten whole
1 crispbread with a little butter

11 AM
1 glass of mineral water

LUNCH
1 small black coffee
4 oz. (125 g) carton of plain cottage cheese
1 fresh orange

TEA-TIME
1 glass of mineral water or 1 cup of tea with lemon only

DINNER
Choose a good portion of *one* of the following (grilled or baked only):

chicken, without the skin
lamb
beef, without fat
liver
veal
fish of any kind

Do remember, no rich sauces or gravy are to accompany any of the above dishes, but you may have a good sized mixed green salad, dressed with a little oil and lemon, salt and pepper.

Plus 1 fresh orange for dessert
1 small black coffee *or* 1 glass of mineral water

You may switch lunch and dinner if you wish.

Two-Week Diets

A two-week diet regime can either be on the basis of one week on/one week off or, for the best results, two whole weeks without breaking the regime. If you are planning a two-week diet, then do ensure beforehand that you have the time and few or no social commitments. Make a determined effort not to give in and the rewards at the end of the two weeks will be well worth it.

YOGHURT DIET
(average weight loss is 11 lb. in two weeks)

Here is a very simple two-week yoghurt diet, which can enable you to lose up to eleven pounds. You follow a simple, two-day eating plan, which you repeat for two weeks, and each day, five times a day, a small carton of yoghurt is included with your food.

Day 1
BREAKFAST
1 small glass of vegetable or tomato juice, with black pepper and Worcestershire sauce
1 boiled egg
1 cup of black coffee or lemon tea
1 natural yoghurt

11 AM
1 natural yoghurt
1 cup of tea or coffee

LUNCH
1 small glass of vegetable or tomato juice
1 yoghurt mixed with *either* 2 tablespoons of fresh fruit salad *or* fresh vegetable salad
1 cup of black coffee or tea with lemon

DINNER
1 cup of any clear soup, with lemon juice and black pepper
1 lightly boiled egg
1 thin slice of wholemeal bread with margarine
1 plain yoghurt
1 small cup of black coffee

BEFORE RETIRING
1 plain yoghurt
1 apple

Day 2
BREAKFAST
1 small glass of tomato juice or vegetable juice
2 crispbreads with butter
1 piece of any fresh fruit
1 cup of tea or coffee
1 plain yoghurt

11 AM
1 cup of tea or coffee
1 piece of fresh fruit

LUNCH
Either a 2-egg omelette with any filling plus a small green salad
Or 6 oz. (175 g) of chicken with a salad made from lettuce, watercress, apple, onion and cucumber, with a little vinegar and oil dressing
Or a grilled cheeseburger made with fresh mince meat and topped with a slice of Edam, Gouda or Cheddar cheese

Plus 1 green vegetable
1 piece of fresh fruit
1 cup of tea or coffee
1 plain yoghurt

DINNER
6 oz. (175 g) of any lean meat or white fish, cooked any way except fried. Try to vary your choice, e.g. if you choose the cheeseburger for lunch then have fish in the evening. Serve with *either* grilled tomatoes *or* a green salad, with a little vinegar and oil dressing, as at lunch.

Plus 1 small black coffee
1 plain yoghurt

Day 3
The same as Day 1

Day 4
The same as Day 2

Continue in this pattern until you have completed your two weeks.

Do not use sugar or milk in tea or coffee, but an artificial sweetener is permitted.

ALTERNATING DIET
(average weight loss 10–12 lb. in two weeks)

This diet is extra high in proteins as well as vitamins and minerals. It will not leave you feeling tired or hungry or lacking in energy. You will notice a difference in your skin and will be brimming over with added vitality.

Day 1: The Meat Day
½ glass of freshly squeezed orange juice
2 eggs, scrambled without milk or fat. Cook in non-stick pan.
1 thin slice wholemeal toast. (Pile eggs onto unbuttered toast.)
1 cup herbal tea or tea with lemon *or* 1 glass of skimmed milk

MID-MORNING
2 sticks of celery eaten with 2 tablespoons of cottage cheese
1 glass of mineral water

LUNCH
4 oz. (125 g) grilled hamburger *or* 4 oz. (125 g) minute steak. Mustard is permitted, but no other sauces.
large green salad with oil and lemon dressing.
1 carton of natural yoghurt plus 1 teaspoon of honey
1 cup of herbal tea or tea with lemon or 1 glass of skimmed milk

TEA-TIME
1 small banana
1 glass mineral water

DINNER
4 oz. (125 g) grilled chicken, turkey, veal or liver
large green salad. Use ½ avocado pear in the salad plus oil and lemon dressing.
½ grapefruit (no sugar)
1 cup of herbal tea or tea with lemon or glass of skimmed milk

Day 2: The Fish Day
BREAKFAST
½ glass freshly squeezed orange juice
4 thin slices of grilled bacon (cook until crisp)
½ grapefruit peeled and segmented
1 thin slice of wholewheat toast. (Pile bacon and grapefruit segments onto unbuttered toast.)
1 cup of herbal tea or tea with lemon or 1 glass of skimmed milk

MID-MORNING
½ banana
1 glass of mineral water

LUNCH
4 oz. (125 g) tuna fish *or* sardines (drain off oil) *or* peeled prawns
large green salad with oil and lemon dressing
½ grapefruit (no sugar)
1 cup of herbal tea or tea with lemon or 1 glass of skimmed milk

TEA-TIME
½ banana
1 glass of mineral water

DINNER
4 oz. (125 g) grilled white fish such as plaice, cod, turbot, haddock, sole, coley
large green salad. Add ½ avocado to the salad, plus oil and lemon dressing.
½ grapefruit (no sugar)
1 cup of herbal tea or tea with lemon or glass of skimmed milk

NB Although grapefruit is normally a starter, with this particular diet I suggest it should be eaten last to refresh the palate.

WONDER DIET
(average weight loss 10–12 lb. in two weeks)

The Wonder Diet could be called a re-education of eating habits as well as aiding better health and replenishing essential minerals and vitamins often lacking after winter. There is ample choice and variation with new tastes and ideas in presentation.

BREAKFAST
You must eat the following every day:

½ grapefruit (no sugar)
1 egg (cooked to your liking)
1 thin slice of wholemeal toast plus a dab of butter or margarine
1 cup of coffee or tea with milk (no sugar but artificial sweetener permitted)

On Saturdays and Sundays you may add:
1 lean slice of grilled bacon
1 grilled tomato
4–5 mushrooms

LUNCH
Every day:
Fresh vegetable and fruit salad. Eat as much as you want, using as many different vegetables and fruit combinations as you like. Here are some examples: green peppers, celery, spring onions and apples; red or white cabbage, cucumber, carrots and grapes; lettuce, onion, red pepper and plums; cauliflower, tomato, leeks and tangerines; Chinese cabbage, grated turnip, mushrooms and oranges.

Method
Finely chop or grate the salad ingredients. Arrange on a large plate. Sprinkle each salad with 1 dessertspoon of chopped nuts and any fresh herbs you can find. If fresh ones are not available then substitute dried ones. Finally make a dressing for your salad using freshly squeezed lemon juice, a little oil and salt and pepper.

Plus 1 glass of mineral water and a small coffee or tea with milk but no sugar

DINNER
Choose one of the following dishes:

Either 4–6 oz. (125–175 g) of steamed, grilled or baked plaice, haddock or cod. (If you grill you may use a small knob of butter. If you bake add a small knob of butter and the juice of half a lemon.)

Or 4–6 oz. (125–175 g) of chicken, turkey, veal, chicken livers or lean mince. (Meat should be grilled or baked with lemon juice or herbs. Chicken livers and mince can be cooked in a non-stick pan using lemon juice and herbs and garlic salt. If you choose the chicken livers, be sure not to overcook them. They should not require longer than 6–8 minutes. Mince may take a little longer.)

2 of the following vegetables: brussels sprouts, carrots, leeks, swede, turnips, parsnips, broccoli, celery, cauliflower, beans, mangetout. (Vegetables should be firm and not overcooked. Use water sparingly and add the juice of ½ a lemon to help flavour, retain colour and add additional vitamin and mineral content.)

1 piece of fresh fruit of your choice. (If you choose grapes then you may have up to 12.)

Plus mineral water followed by 1 small coffee *or* tea with milk but no sugar

DOROTHY'S ONION DIET
(average weight loss 10–12 lb. in two weeks)

My girl friend Dorothy had this marvellous diet given to her by a Turkish doctor. The diet is taken in the form of a soup, which is designed to help the body release toxins and waste products, thereby cleansing the blood and improving the circulation. Dorothy suggests that the soup should be kept in a vacuum flask to retain its heat. This way, the soup, always taken hot, fills you up easily. If you prefer a thin soup to a thickish purée, you simply add more hot water.

Here is the recipe for one day's supply of onion soup:

8 large onions
2 lb. of any other two vegetables (e.g. 1 lb. runner beans plus 1 lb. marrow; *or* 1 lb. cabbage plus 1 lb. cauliflower). The only other vegetables you cannot use are carrots, tomatoes or potatoes.

Method
Chop up onions into smallish chunks. Place in large saucepan and cover with 2½ pints of cold water. Add 1 meat stock cube and some freshly ground pepper. Bring to the boil and cook for 3–4 minutes only. Remove vegetables. Do not throw away the water, but keep it hot. Pass vegetables through a blender or liquidiser, or mash with a potato masher. Then return vegetables to the water and stir well. Pour into a vacuum flask and it is ready to eat.

Here, then, is the diet:

Day 1
Eat any fresh fruit – except bananas – for breakfast, lunch and dinner in any quantity. Take your onion soup throughout the day. You may have up to 3 cups of herbal tea only, or tea with lemon, but no coffee.

Day 2
For breakfast have your soup and a cup of tea. For lunch and dinner eat mixed green salads only, dressed with lemon juice and pepper. Drink your soup throughout the day. You may have 2 further cups of tea if you want them, either herbal or with lemon only.

Day 3
For breakfast, lunch, and dinner mix fresh fruit (except bananas) and green salads together as a meal, or eat them separately. Take the soup throughout the day plus up to 3 cups of tea if you need them.

Day 4
BREAKFAST
1 cup of onion soup, plus, if you wish, a cup of tea as before.

LUNCH
1 chicken breast (the chicken must be boiled only.) Don't forget to have your soup throughout the day. You may have tea as before.

Day 5
For one whole day you may have 12 oz. (350 g) of any fat-free meat, grilled only. Plus 5 tomatoes, grilled or raw. Remember to divide the meat and tomatoes into three meals. Have your soup throughout the day and your 3 cups of tea as before.

Day 6
Today you may have as much fat-free meat as you want. (You are not restricted to 12 oz. (350 g) as yesterday.) You may also have a mixed green salad with your meat meals. Don't forget to drink your soup throughout the day and you may have your 3 cups of tea as before.

Day 7
Breakfast, lunch and dinner: eat only 3 tablespoons of plain boiled rice at each meal, mixed into your onion soup. To drink, you may have fresh fruit juice throughout the day and remember your onion soup in between meals as well.

Days 8–14
Repeat as for days 1–7.

PAINLESS DIET
(average weight loss 10–12 lb. in two weeks)

This diet has been designed for simplicity and ease. There is no cooking involved and you should not exceed your normal food budget. Breakfast and supper are light meals, with a hearty salad full of natural goodness for lunch.

BREAKFAST
For your health cup you will need:

½ punnet of fresh strawberries *or* one tablespoon of finely chopped uncooked rhubarb
¼ bunch watercress
1 small carton natural yoghurt
2 tablespoons cottage cheese
1 small finely grated carrot
½ teaspoon freshly chopped mint
½ teaspoon freshly chopped parsley

Method
Put ingredients into a liquidiser for about 30 seconds, then pour into a tall glass and drink immediately. (If you do not have a liquidiser, mash and whisk together with a hand whisk the yoghurt and cottage cheese.) Add carrot. Chop watercress, including stalks, together with mint and parsley and mix these with yoghurt and cottage cheese. Pour mixture over strawberries or rhubarb in a glass bowl. It is then ready to eat.

Plus 1 cup of lemon or herbal tea

LUNCH
Midday health salad made with the following:

1 thinly sliced orange
2 oz. (50 g) nuts of your choice (crumbled)
1 small carrot
4–5 young dandelion leaves (optional)
3 radishes
3–4 mangetouts (if not available, use 1 tablespoon raw, fresh young peas)
4–5 endive leaves or chicory
rest of watercress from breakfast
fresh herbs

Method
Arrange ingredients attractively on a dish, then sprinkle on the nuts and finely chopped herbs. Mix 1 tablespoon of olive oil and 1 tablespoon of lemon juice with a pinch of mustard powder and black pepper. Pour over the salad and it is ready to eat.

Plus 1 cup of lemon or herbal tea

DINNER
This is a light snack. Combine together 1 small carton of natural yoghurt, 2 tablespoons of cottage cheese, 1 dessertspoon of honey, 1 tablespoon of raisins and ¼ teaspoon each of powdered ginger and cinnamon.

Plus 1 cup of lemon or herbal tea

Throughout the day you may have, in addition, up to 3 glasses of water or fruit juice with this diet.

REVITALISING DIET
(average weight loss 10–12 lb. in two weeks)

My revitalising diet will make you feel so good, so clean and so light, that you will be tempted to try it over and over again. To make each meal different and delicious, choose widely from my list. Do not eat the same vegetables and fruit every day: boredom is the slimmer's worst enemy.

ON RISING
1 small glass of hot water plus juice of ½ lemon

BREAKFAST
Beat together in a tall glass:

½ pint skimmed or low-fat milk
1 fresh egg
1 teaspoon honey

Drink this in place of breakfast.

Plus you may have one of the following:

1 apple
1 pear
½ melon
10–12 grapes
3–4 plums

MID-MORNING
1 cup of tea with lemon (no sugar)

LUNCH
This is taken as a large salad, eating as much as you want to fill you up, choosing vegetables from the following:

Lettuce, cucumber, watercress, courgettes, mustard and cress, mushrooms, endive, beetroot, chicory, bean sprouts, spring onions, celery, cauliflower, carrots, snow peas (mangetout), green or red peppers.

Remember to choose at least four different ones from the list for each salad and all vegetables must be eaten raw. For the dressing use oil/lemon or oil/vinegar and some fresh herbs. If you cannot find fresh ones then you may substitute dried ones.

Method
Put the dressing and herbs in a salad bowl together and allow them to marinate for about five minutes, then toss in the vegetables and mix thoroughly.

Plus 1 large glass of mineral water

TEA-TIME
1 cup of tea with lemon (no sugar)

DINNER
Mix together in a tall glass:
¼ pint skimmed or low-fat milk
¼ pint tomato juice
1 teaspoon Worcester sauce
2 teaspoons finely chopped parsley
2 teaspoons finely chopped nuts

Drink this in place of a meal.

Plus 1 banana and 1 glass of mineral water

BOOSTER DIET
(average weight loss 10–12 lb. in two weeks)

The Booster Diet is simple and will not burn a hole in your purse either! The ingredients are all essential for good health and will not leave you feeling hungry. This diet is followed on the basis of three days on and one day off for two weeks. On days off, keep to a light sensible eating plan.

Day 1
BREAKFAST
1 small carton of natural yoghurt
1 fresh egg
1 teaspoon of honey
1 teaspoon of bran
1 teaspoon of chopped nuts

Method
Beat the egg, add yoghurt, honey and bran and beat all together. Serve in a glass bowl with nuts sprinkled on top.

Plus 1 cup of tea with lemon (only artificial sweetener permitted) or a herbal tea such as mint

LUNCH
1 large carton natural yoghurt
1 small apple, unpeeled but finely chopped
6 grapes cut in half
1 stick of celery, finely chopped
½ bunch of watercress
½ lemon
salt and pepper to taste

DINNER
Same as breakfast

Day 2
BREAKFAST
1 small carton of natural yoghurt
1 small banana
1 orange or tangerine or satsuma
1 teaspoon of honey
1 teaspoon of bran

Method
Chop up fruit, mix yoghurt, honey and bran together and then pour over fruit.

Plus 1 cup of tea as for Day One

LUNCH
1 large carton of natural yoghurt
4 oz. (125 g) of cold chicken or turkey or shrimps
½ cucumber
1 spring onion
½ teaspoon of curry powder
1 teaspoon of tomato sauce
juice of a lemon
2–3 celery tops

Method
Dice up meat or shrimps, plus cucumber and spring onion. Place in a bowl and mix tomato sauce, curry powder, lemon juice with yoghurt. Pour over meat or fish, toss well and serve on a bed of celery tops.

Plus 1 cup of tea as for Day One

DINNER
1 small carton of natural yoghurt
1 pear
½ melon
1 teaspoon of honey
1 teaspoon of bran
½ teaspoonful of ground ginger

Method
Chop up pear and melon, mix honey and bran with yoghurt. Pour over fruit, and sprinkle with ginger.

Plus 1 cup of tea as for Day One

Day 3
BREAKFAST
1 small carton of natural yoghurt
6 prunes and 4 apricots (use these either dried or soaked)
1 teaspoon of honey
1 teaspoon of bran

Method
Chop up prunes and apricots and place in a bowl. Mix honey and bran with yoghurt and pour over fruit.

Plus 1 cup of tea as for Day One

LUNCH
1 small carton of natural yoghurt
¼ of an iceberg lettuce (or the equivalent of Chinese cabbage)
½ melon left over from yesterday
5–6 raw mushrooms
½ lemon
salt and pepper to taste
1 egg, hard boiled
½ bunch of watercress (from yesterday)

Method
Chop lettuce, melon and raw mushrooms and place in a bowl together. Mix the juice from the lemon with the yoghurt, plus salt and pepper to taste and pour over the fruit and vegetables. On a separate plate, serve the hard boiled egg, cut into quarters on a bed of watercress with the yoghurt salad.

Plus 1 cup of tea as for Day One

DINNER
1 small carton of natural yoghurt
2 passion fruit *or* 2 fresh figs *or* 4–5 dates
1 teaspoon of honey
1 teaspoon of bran

Method
Prepare and chop up fruit. Place in a bowl, mix honey and bran into yoghurt and pour over fruit.

Plus 1 cup of tea as for Day One

Three-Week Diets

Diets of this length are ideal before a summer holiday, and give you time to get yourself into shape – you will feel younger and much better for it. It's probably a good idea to follow a diet together with your partner. But if you want to lose weight and he does not, then include him in just a few meals. This will at least help to re-educate his eating habits.

MONDAY TO FRIDAY DIET
(average weight loss 12–15 lb. in three weeks)

On this diet you eat every two hours with plenty of choice. The Monday to Friday Diet is the answer for people who can only socialise at weekends, because on this diet you're only following the regime from Monday to Friday. However, it would be unwise to go 'mad' at the weekends. Be sensible and the diet will work.

Here is an example of a typical day's menu taken from the choice of dishes available every two hours:

8 AM
1 glass of fresh orange juice
6 prunes
2 tablespoons of yoghurt

10 AM
1 Ryvita with a smear of butter and honey
1 cup of coffee or tea

MID-DAY
2 slices of cold chicken
some slices of cucumber
1 teaspoonful of sweet pickle

2 PM
2 finger-size wedges of cheese
1 tangerine

4 PM
1 digestive biscuit
1 cup of coffee or tea

6 PM
1 grilled hamburger
3 grilled tomatoes

8 PM
1 small bunch of black grapes
1 glass of water

Three-Week Diets

10 PM
1 tablespoon of mixed nuts and raisins
1 cup of coffee or tea

For good results do not repeat foods on the same day. If you choose a digestive biscuit at 4 p.m. don't have another at 10 p.m. If you feel you don't want to eat as often as every two hours, then that is entirely up to you. But for most slimmers, hunger pangs and variety are what matter most and breakfast is a must.

Here then is the diet:

8 AM (first meal choice)
Either mix together in a tall glass and drink:

1 glass fresh fruit juice
2 teaspoons wheatgerm
1 teaspoon of honey
Or 1 glass fruit juice
6 prunes
2 tablespoons of natural yoghurt
Or 1 glass fruit juice
2 tablespoons cottage cheese
4 segments of grapefruit
Or 1 glass fruit juice
1 whole orange
Or 1 glass fruit juice
1 whole grapefruit
Or 1 glass fruit juice
2 tablespoons stewed apple

Plus 1 cup of herbal tea or tea with lemon or black coffee (no sugar)

10 AM (second meal choice)
Either 1 Ryvita with smear of butter and honey
Or 1 boiled egg plus ½ slice of wholewheat toast with smear of butter
Or 1 thin slice of ham
1 slice pineapple
Or 1 poached egg
1 Ryvita with smear of butter
Or 1 thin slice of wholemeal bread with smear of butter covered with thin slice of Cheddar cheese
Or 1 tablespoon of muesli cereal with a little milk (no sugar)

Plus 1 cup of coffee or tea with milk (no sugar)

MID-DAY
Either mixed green salad topped with thinly sliced small banana and a little French dressing
Or 2 medium carrots grated, 1 stick of celery grated and mixed together with 1 tablespoon of mixed nuts and a little French dressing
Or 2 slices of lean cold chicken or turkey with 1 teaspoon of sweet pickle and some sliced cucumber
Or 1 tablespoon of sweetcorn, hot or cold, mixed with 1 tablespoon of chopped red or green peppers and 1 tablespoon flaked almonds
Or 2 tablespoons well-drained tuna fish served on a bed of lettuce with a wedge of lemon

Plus 1 glass of mineral water

2 PM (fourth meal choice)
Either 1 apple or orange or pear
Or 1 tablespoon salted peanuts
Or 1 fruit yoghurt
Or 3–4 pieces of dried fruit such as apricots, apples, plums or prunes to be eaten raw
Or 1 tablespoon of cottage cheese with a few slices of cucumber
Or a 2-finger wedge of cheese with 1 tangerine

Plus 1 cup of tea with lemon or 1 black coffee (no sugar)

4 PM (fifth meal choice)
Either 2 tablespoons fresh fruit salad
Or 1 large stick of celery filled with cottage cheese
Or 1 thick slice of apple spread with honey
Or 1 dry cracker spread with Marmite and a few thin slices of cucumber
Or ½ a slice of wholewheat toast spread with a smear of butter
Or 1 digestive biscuit

Plus 1 cup of tea or coffee with milk (no sugar)

6 PM (sixth meal choice)
Either 2-egg omelette stuffed with chopped mushrooms cooked in a non-stick pan

Or 1 grilled hamburger and 3 grilled tomatoes

Or 1 medium-sized jacket potato stuffed with cottage cheese and chopped parsley

Or 2 medium fillets of plaice or haddock or coley or sole, poached in milk and water or grilled with lemon juice and served with 1 tablespoon of boiled carrots

Or 2 slices of grilled liver served with a green salad and a little French dressing

Or 1 bowl of vegetable broth made from fresh vegetables. Just before serving add 1 raw egg.

Plus 1 glass of mineral water

8 PM (seventh meal choice)

Either ½ grapefruit sprinkled with a little blackcurrant juice and cinnamon and grilled for 3–4 minutes

Or 1 fresh peach

Or 1 small bunch of white grapes

Or 1 slice of melon

Or 1 natural yoghurt with cinnamon and some raisins added

Or a portion of any stewed fruit (no sugar)

Plus 1 small cup of black coffee or 1 glass of water

10 PM (eighth meal choice)
Either 1 digestive biscuit
Or 1 tablespoon of mixed nuts and raisins
Or 1 slice of melon
Or 1 thin slice of wholewheat toast with a little butter

Plus a night cap of a milky coffee or tea or 1 cup of herbal tea

TRY ME DIET
(average weight loss 12–15 lb. in three weeks)

This diet is followed on a pattern of 3 days on, 2 days off for three weeks. The main ingredients are all readily available and the dishes should appeal to you at any time to add zest to meat or fish dishes on non-diet days.

BREAKFAST
A good portion of stewed apple sprinkled with cinnamon and chopped nuts
1 thin slice of wholewheat toast spread with a little butter and smear of honey

Plus 1 cup of herbal tea or tea with lemon (no milk or sugar)

MID-MORNING
1 glass mineral water or fresh fruit juice

LUNCH
A mixed salad made from 1 cup of grated fresh carrots, 1 cup of grated fresh turnip, 1 tablespoonful of mixed nuts, 1 tablespoon of raisins

Method
Mix salad ingredients together and add 2 tablespoonsful of dressing made from lemon juice, white vinegar, and some chopped herbs. Mix together and pour over the salad.

Plus 1 starch-reduced crispbread, 1 cup of herbal tea or tea with lemon

TEA-TIME
1 glass of mineral water or fresh fruit juice

DINNER
A ginger health platter:
1 large cooking apple, diced
1 large or 2 medium carrots
½ turnip

This quantity should fill approximately 2 medium teacups.

1 small onion, chopped
1" of fresh ginger or 1 flat teaspoonful of powdered ginger

The ginger adds zest and flavour to the dish; also many people swear by it for the cure and prevention of colds and flu. But if you don't like ginger, simply leave it out.

2 tablespoons of cold, cooked meat, diced (any left-over meat will do)

Method
In a medium saucepan or, better still, a wok, fry the onion, ginger and meat together in 1 tablespoonful of oil until the onions become transparent. Then, using a wooden spoon, toss in the rest of the ingredients. Cook over rapid heat for about 5 minutes. Then add the juice of 1 lemon, freshly ground black pepper, and cook for a further 3 minutes. Serve hot on a large plate, sprinkled with chopped fresh parsley.

Plus 1 cup of herbal tea or tea with lemon or 1 glass of mineral water

SHERRY DIET
(average weight loss 12–15lb. in three weeks)

This diet includes a glass of sherry every evening and can be followed on work days only, leaving the weekends free to eat healthfully and sensibly. If followed for three weeks on a Monday to Friday basis, the average weight loss over three weeks is about 12–15 lb.

BREAKFAST
1 medium glass of tomato juice to which has been added 1 heaped teaspoon of wheatgerm. Mix together and drink.
1 thin slice of wholemeal bread, plain or toasted, spread with 1 teaspoon of honey (no butter or margarine). Add 1 slice of hard cheese cut to the same size as the bread.

Plus 1 cup of tea with lemon or milk (no sugar)

LUNCH
Salad: ingredients for this are:
3–4 kinds of fresh winter vegetables (preferably including fresh spinach, mushrooms or onions), diced
1 dessertspoon of sliced almonds
1 dessertspoon of peanut butter
juice from 1 lemon
1 orange
1 tablespoon of parmesan or other hard cheese
1 teaspoon of finely chopped fresh herbs of your choice
1 tablespoon of finely grated fresh breadcrumbs

Method
Put all the diced vegetables into a fairly large saucepan. Add the orange and lemon juice and some salt and pepper to taste. Put on a high heat and cook quickly, tossing the vegetables for approximately 3 minutes.

Remove and place the vegetables and the remaining juice in a suitable fireproof dish. Spread the peanut butter over the top of the vegetables, then add the sliced almonds and finally the cheese, breadcrumbs and herbs, mixed together, to make a top layer.

Place under a hot grill till well toasted on top. Serve with a wedge of lemon.

Dessert: 1 piece of fresh fruit of your choice

Plus 1 glass of tomato juice, or tea with lemon or milk (no sugar)

DINNER
Blend or beat well together with a hand whisk the following ingredients, and drink:

½ pint of tomato juice
1 small glass of sherry (dry or sweet)
2 teaspoons of parsley, finely chopped
2 tablespoons of yoghurt
1 fresh egg

BEFORE RETIRING
1 cup of tea with lemon or milk (no sugar)

THREE BY THREE DIET
(average weight loss 12–15 lb. in three weeks)

The title of this diet describes exactly what you do: three days on and three days off. Non-diet days are to be followed by eating sensibly, avoiding those foods you know are fattening.

For three days' supply you will need:
1½ lb. of blackcurrants
1½ lb. rhubarb
4 tablespoons of honey
½ teaspoonful of cinnamon powder
juice from 4 large oranges
4 tablespoons of water

For fruit compote:
Gently bring to the boil all the ingredients together, then allow to simmer for approximately five minutes. Remove from the heat and cool. Store in a large bowl, cover with foil, and place in the bottom of the fridge.

BREAKFAST
3–4 tablespoons of fruit compote
Plus 1 glass of mineral water or 1 cup of herbal tea or tea with lemon

MID-MORNING
1 glass of mineral water or 1 cup of herbal tea or tea with lemon
Plus 1 fresh orange

LUNCH
3–4 tablespoons of fruit compote
1 small carton of cottage cheese
1 starch-reduced crispbread

Plus 1 glass of mineral water or 1 cup of herbal tea or tea with lemon

TEA-TIME
1 glass of mineral water or 1 cup of herbal tea or tea with lemon

Plus 1 fresh orange

DINNER
3–4 tablespoons of fruit compote
3 oz. (75 g) of any hard cheese
1 dry starch-reduced crispbread

Plus 1 cup of herbal tea, or tea with lemon, or 1 glass of mineral water

BEFORE RETIRING
1 glass of mineral water
1 fresh orange

MY HIGH FIBRE DIET
(average weight loss 12–15 lb. in three weeks)

What is the best and cheapest way of introducing fibre to the family diet without incurring additional cost? The answer is to eat raw at least one complete meal a day, but ideally a little with each meal is far better. This diet will show you how.

Mixing raw fruits and vegetables gives higher fibre intake and, if you can add 2 slices of wholemeal or rye bread a day and some nuts, your fibre intake will be considerably improved.

To make the idea of fibre intake even more appealing, here is my own home-made combination which I call my high fibre mix. This should be taken four times a day with meals.

To make the mix sufficient for one day, you need:
2 tablespoons of rough porridge oats
1 teaspoon of walnuts and hazelnuts (coarsely chopped) or pine kernels (do not crush these)
1 teaspoon of toasted rice grains

Method
Mix the oats with the nuts or pine kernels. Put raw rice grains into a heated dry pan and toast over a medium heat till golden brown. Mix rice with oats and nuts.

This delicious nutty mixture can be sprinkled over vegetable salads, added to raw fruit salads, or mixed with natural yoghurts, and you can combine it with small amounts (about ½ a teaspoon) of golden syrup to make high-fibre sweet chews, which you can eat as a snack, but not more than four a day!

To make sure you choose the right high fibre vegetables, here is a list to choose from:

Broccoli, Brussels sprouts, cabbage, cauliflower, beetroot, carrots, tomatoes, aubergines, marrow, radishes and spinach.

Here is a list of summer fruits to choose from:

strawberries, cherries, black, red and white currants, raspberries, plums, peaches, greengages, apples and pears.

For maximum fibre do not remove skin. Here are three delicious 'mix and match' fruit and vegetable combination salads which could be taken as a complete meal or as an accompaniment to cheese, eggs, meat or fish:

(i) Strawberries, plums, almonds, hazelnuts, tomatoes, cauliflower, lettuce, plus any fresh herbs such as basil, dill or parsley. Arrange these attractively on a plate and dress with a little oil and lemon.

(ii) Cherries, any mixed nuts including salted peanuts, beetroot, and celery (plus tops). Arrange on a large plate and dress with fresh herbs mixed with a little cider vinegar.

(iii) Red currants, peaches, apricots, cherries, beetroot, radishes, almonds, grated carrots and fresh spinach. Arrange on a large plate and dress with a little oil and lemon.

Now here is a suggested 5-day eating plan for you to follow to aid weight loss and improve your health:

BREAKFAST
1 glass of hot water to which the juice of 1 fresh orange has been added
1 bowl of natural yoghurt mixed with 2 tablespoons of high-fibre mix
1 thin slice of wholemeal or rye bread smeared with a little butter

Plus 1 cup of herbal tea or tea with lemon

MID-MORNING
1 glass of mineral water or fresh fruit juice

LUNCH
A large salad from my 'mix and match' combination
1 glass of mineral water or fresh fruit juice

TEA-TIME
1 cup of herbal tea or tea with lemon (no sugar)
1–2 high-fibre sweet chews

DINNER
Small portion of grilled meat, or grilled fish, or cheese or eggs
'Mix and match' salad
1 thin slice of wholemeal or rye bread with a smear of butter
1 piece of fresh fruit

Plus 1 glass of mineral water

DAY BY DAY DIET
(average weight loss 12–15 lb. in three weeks)

This diet is so easy because it is followed on a day on, day off basis. At the end of three weeks not only will your weight loss have improved, but your whole body will be revitalised. Remember, 'off days' are sensible days!

On diet days:
ON RISING
1 glass of hot water with 2 slices of orange added

BREAKFAST
1 whole orange or 1 whole grapefruit

Plus 1 glass of mineral water and 1 small cup of herbal tea

MID-MORNING
1 glass of hot water to which is added 2 slices of orange

LUNCH
1 carrot (finely grated)
1 stick of celery (finely grated)
1 apple (finely grated)

Sprinkle the above ingredients with lemon and fresh herbs.

Plus 1 glass of hot water with 2 slices of orange added

DINNER
portion of freshly cooked spinach (cook only for 2 minutes in very little water and sprinkle with lemon juice and fresh herbs)
small bowl of fresh fruit salad

Plus 1 glass of mineral water

BEFORE RETIRING
1 cup of herbal tea

WINTER FLAB DIET
(average weight loss 12–15 lb. in three weeks)

If you feel in need of a pick-me-up diet, to rid yourself of all that winter flab accumulation, then this diet might be the answer. The routine is not difficult, since the pattern of the diet is four days on and four days off.

BREAKFAST
Mix together the following ingredients:
1 cup of natural yoghurt
½ an orange (chopped into segments)
½ a grapefruit
3 chopped dates
1 tablespoon of rosehip syrup (available at all chemists)

MID-MORNING
Mix together the following to make a yoghurt cup:
1 glass of mineral water
1 cup of natural yoghurt
juice of ½ lemon
black pepper to taste

LUNCH
1 avocado (cut in half with the stone removed)
1 orange or 2 tangerines (chopped)
1 oz. (25 g) almonds (chopped)
2 tablespoons of natural yoghurt

Method
Combine the fruit, nuts and yoghurt and fill each half of the avocado with the mixture. Serve on a bed of freshly chopped celery tops.

Plus A wedge of lemon, 2 sticks of celery, 1 glass of mineral water, and 1 cup of herbal tea with lemon

TEA-TIME
Same as mid-morning

DINNER

4–6 oz. (125–175 g) (depending on your appetite) of peeled shrimps or finely chopped cooked chicken, served on a bed of fresh watercress (use a whole bunch) and 4 or 5 thinly sliced mushrooms.

Serve with a dressing made from 4 tablespoons of natural yoghurt, the juice of 1 fresh lemon, plus (if you like it) 1 clove of freshly crushed garlic.

Dessert:
1 fresh pear or a small bunch of grapes

Plus 1 glass of mineral water and 1 cup of herbal tea with lemon

Four-Week Diets

At the end of a whole month of dieting you should feel like a new person, determined not to let yourself slip back into those old habits. What was once a life-long problem has been overcome and it is up to you to maintain those good results. If ever you are weak willed or over-indulge on a weekend, put yourself back onto a one-or two-day incentive diet to get rid of those few pounds quickly, before they have time to accumulate. Then continue on a sensible, well-balanced eating programme.

HUNGRY MAN'S DIET
(average weight loss 20–28 lb. in four weeks)

This man's diet I designed with plenty of variation, using food that was both sustaining and satisfying. For the really over-weight, the first two days are going to need the most will-power, but, once overcome, the rest is easy.

Day 1
BREAKFAST
1 fresh orange, to be eaten whole
1 cup of tea or coffee, with milk but no sugar
1 crispbread with butter
1 oz. (25 g) of Edam or Cheddar cheese

MID-MORNING
1 large glass of hot water and the juice of 2 lemons sweetened with 1 teaspoon honey

LUNCH
2-egg omelette, served with 3 grilled tomatoes
1 small cup of black coffee or tea with lemon, no sugar

TEA-TIME
1 fresh orange, to be eaten whole

DINNER
4–6 good-sized slices of cold chicken, no skin. Serve with a salad of 2 sticks of celery, watercress and cucumber. No salad dressing or pickles, but you can have mustard.
1 small cup of black coffee or tea with lemon, no sugar

Day 2
BREAKFAST
½ a grapefruit with ½ a teaspoon of sugar
1 boiled egg
1 crispbread with butter
1 cup of coffee or tea with milk, but no sugar

MID-MORNING
1 large glass of hot water and the juice of 2 lemons, sweetened with 1 teaspoon of honey

LUNCH
3 slices of corned beef
2 tablespoons of runner beans
2 crispbreads with 1 oz. (25 g) of Edam or Cheddar cheese
1 small cup of black coffee, no sugar

TEA-TIME
½ a grapefruit with ½ a teaspoon of sugar

DINNER
1 bowl of tomato soup
4 oz. (125 g) grated Edam or Cheddar cheese, served with a good-sized mixed salad, using what vegetables you like. No salad cream, but you may have a dressing of 1 dessertspoon of oil and 2 dessertspoons of lemon juice.
1 small cup of black coffee or tea with lemon, no sugar

Day 3
BREAKFAST
6–8 prunes, mixed with 1 chopped apple and 1 tablespoon of muesli or similar cereal
1 cup of coffee or tea with milk, but no sugar

MID-MORNING
1 large glass of hot water with the juice of 2 lemons and 1 teaspoon of honey

LUNCH
3 lean slices of hot or cold roast beef, with 2 tablespoons of broccoli
1 pear or 1 apple
1 small cup of black coffee, no sugar

TEA-TIME
1 cup of tea with milk, no sugar
1 crispbread with butter
1 oz. (25 g) of Edam or Cheddar cheese

DINNER
1 boiled egg
1 crispbread with butter
1 bowl of fresh fruit salad
1 small cup of black coffee, no sugar

Day 4
BREAKFAST
1 bowl of stewed apples, sweetened with honey
2 lean slices of grilled bacon, no fat
1 poached egg
1 small cup of black coffee or tea with lemon, no sugar

MID-MORNING
1 large glass of hot water with the juice of 2 lemons, sweetened with 1 teaspoon of honey

LUNCH
2 crispbreads with butter, topped with 2 oz. (50 g) of Edam or Cheddar cheese, tomato, onion and cucumber
1 small cup of black coffee, no sugar

TEA-TIME
1 fresh apple

DINNER
2 lean, grilled lamb cutlets. Serve with as many grilled mushrooms and grilled tomatoes as you want, 1 tablespoon of cauliflower and salt, pepper and mustard.
1 small cup of black coffee, no sugar

Day 5
BREAKFAST
1 fresh orange
2 eggs, scrambled
1 crispbread with butter
1 cup of coffee or tea with milk, no sugar

MID-MORNING
1 glass of hot water with the juice of 2 lemons, sweetened with 1 teaspoon of honey

LUNCH
3 tablespoons of meat casserole, served with 2 tablespoons of any green vegetable, except peas
1 average helping of fresh pineapple or tinned pineapple if you have not got fresh
1 small cup of black coffee, no sugar

TEA-TIME
1 average helping of pineapple

DINNER
3 crispbreads with butter
1 oz. (25 g) of Edam or
1 oz. (25 g) of Gouda
1 fresh orange
1 small black coffee, no sugar

Day 6
BREAKFAST
1 bowl of fresh fruit salad, sprinkled with 1 tablespoon of muesli, or similar cereal
1 cup of coffee or tea with milk, no sugar

MID-MORNING
1 glass of hot water with the juice of two lemons, sweetened with 1 teaspoon of honey

LUNCH
2 grilled sausages with mustard
1 boiled potato
1 tablespoon of broccoli
1 fruit yoghurt
1 small black coffee, no sugar

TEA-TIME
1 bowl of fresh fruit salad

DINNER
1 portion of grilled fish, not silver fish, with lemon. Serve with a mixed green salad, with oil and lemon dressing.
1 crispbread with 1 oz. (25 g) of Edam or Cheddar cheese
1 small black coffee, no sugar

Day 7
BREAKFAST
1 crispbread with butter and honey
1 cup of coffee or tea with milk

MID-MORNING
1 small whisky, if really necessary

LUNCH
Roast meat, no fat, with 1 roast potato and as much as you want of any green vegetable. You may have a little gravy, but no Yorkshire pudding.
1 bowl of fresh fruit salad, with a small portion of ice-cream
If no whisky is taken before lunch, you may have 1 glass of wine.

TEA-TIME
1 cup of tea with lemon

DINNER
2-egg omelette
1 piece of fresh fruit
1 oz. (25 g) of Edam or Cheddar cheese
1 small black coffee, no sugar

The second, third and fourth weeks are the same as the first.

MONDAY TO SUNDAY DIET
(average weight loss 10 lb. in four weeks)

This is a very varied diet, which I have designed to prevent boredom. It is not an expensive diet and one that the whole family could do together.

Monday
BREAKFAST
1 boiled egg
½ a slice of wholemeal bread and butter
1 cup of tea or coffee, without sugar

LUNCH
1 small portion of fish, steamed or grilled, served with 1 small portion of peas
1 piece of fresh fruit
1 glass of milk or 1 cup of tea or coffee, without sugar

DINNER
1 portion of chicken casserole, served with 1 small portion of green salad
½ a slice of wholemeal bread without butter
1 piece of fresh fruit
1 cup of tea or coffee, no sugar

Tuesday
BREAKFAST
1 scrambled egg
½ a slice of wholemeal bread, toasted with butter
1 cup of tea or coffee, no sugar

LUNCH
1 portion of boiled cauliflower with cheese sauce
1 piece of fresh fruit
1 glass of milk or 1 cup of tea or coffee, no sugar

DINNER
1 portion of grilled liver or ham, served with boiled spinach or cabbage
1 small piece of fresh fruit

Wednesday
BREAKFAST
1 slice of wholemeal bread, toasted with butter
1 cup of tea or coffee, no sugar

LUNCH
2-egg plain omelette
1 starch-reduced crispbread
1 piece of fresh fruit
1 glass of milk or 1 cup of tea or coffee, no sugar

DINNER
1 bowl of clear soup
1 grilled steak, served with green boiled vegetables
1 piece of fresh fruit
1 cup of tea or coffee, no sugar

Thursday
BREAKFAST
1 starch-reduced crispbread with butter
1 cup of tea or coffee, no sugar

LUNCH
Grilled fish, served with a green salad
1 piece of fresh fruit
1 cup of tea or coffee, no sugar

DINNER
1 bowl of clear soup
1 grilled steak, served with green boiled vegetables
1 cup of tea or coffee, no sugar

Friday
BREAKFAST
1 boiled egg
½ a slice of wholemeal bread, toasted with butter
1 cup of tea or coffee, no sugar

LUNCH
1 slice of gammon, served with braised celery
1 carton of natural yoghurt *or* 1 piece of fruit
1 glass of milk or 1 cup of tea or coffee, no sugar

DINNER
Poached haddock and egg with grilled tomatoes
1 piece of fresh fruit

Saturday
BREAKFAST
1 scrambled egg on 1 slice of toasted wholemeal bread
1 glass of fruit juice
1 cup of tea or coffee, no sugar

LUNCH
1 bowl of clear soup
cold meat and a green salad
1 slice of melon
1 cup of tea or coffee, no sugar

DINNER
1 portion of meat casserole, served with Brussels sprouts and peas
1 piece of fresh fruit
1 glass of milk or 1 cup of tea or coffee, no sugar

Sunday
BREAKFAST
1 egg, any way you want
1 starch-reduced crispbread
1 small glass of fruit juice
1 cup of tea or coffee, no sugar

LUNCH
1 portion of roast lamb, beef or chicken, served with green boiled vegetables and, if required, 1 small potato
1 piece of fresh fruit
1 cup of tea or coffee, no sugar

DINNER
1 portion of cold meat or chicken, served with 1 medium portion of peas
1 piece of fresh fruit
1 cup of tea or coffee, no sugar

The second, third and fourth weeks are the same as the first.

SECRETARY'S DIET
(average weight loss 15–20 lb. in four weeks)

All secretaries need to keep fit and trim, not only because it improves the looks, but also because the mind is certainly far more alert if you are healthy and fit.

Day 1
BREAKFAST
1 whole grapefruit
1 slimmer's crispbread
1 slice of Edam or Cheddar cheese
1 cup of black coffee

MID-MORNING
1 glass of any kind of fruit juice
1 glass of mineral water

LUNCH
Make a slimmer's open sandwich with 1 thin slice of wholemeal bread. Cover with either 4–6 oz. (125–175 g) of cold chicken, no skin, or 3 oz. (75 g) lean slices of ham or 3 slices of liver sausage. Add 1 tomato and some lettuce and 1 slice of Gouda or Cheddar cheese.

Plus 1 glass of fruit juice

TEA-TIME
1 glass of tea with lemon

DINNER
2-egg omelette. Serve with 1 tablespoon of runner beans and 2 tablespoons of fried mushrooms
1 fresh orange
1 small black coffee

BEFORE RETIRING
1 large glass of mineral water

Day 2
BREAKFAST
1 bowl of stewed prunes with 2 tablespoons of apricots
1 black coffee

MID-MORNING
1 glass of apple juice or mineral water

LUNCH
Make 2 slimmer's open sandwiches with 2 thin slices of wholemeal bread and a little butter. Cover with lettuce, cucumber and watercress.

Plus a slice of melon
1 black coffee

TEA-TIME
Tea with lemon

DINNER
2 lean grilled cutlets. Serve with 2 grilled tomatoes and a small mixed green salad
1 fruit yoghurt
1 glass of apple juice
1 black coffee

BEFORE RETIRING
1 large glass of mineral water

Day 3
BREAKFAST
1 natural yoghurt, mixed with 1 teaspoon of honey
1 fresh orange
1 cup of black coffee

MID-MORNING
1 glass of tomato juice or mineral water

LUNCH
Make 1 slimmer's open sandwich with 1 slice of wholemeal bread and a scraping of butter. Cover with 2 hard-boiled eggs and watercress mixed with chopped apple.

Plus 1 fresh peach or any seasonal fruit
1 small black coffee

TEA-TIME
Tea with lemon

DINNER
6 oz. (175 g) white fish, baked, grilled or fried, served with a mixed green salad
1 fresh apple
2 oz. (50 g) of Edam or Cheddar cheese
1 small black coffee

BEFORE RETIRING
1 glass of mineral water

Day 4
BREAKFAST
1 whole fresh orange
2 crispbreads with a little butter and honey
1 black coffee

MID-MORNING
1 glass of apple juice or mineral water

LUNCH
A slimmer's salad made with ham, Cheddar, Gouda or Edam cheese and a green salad
1 piece of seasonal fruit
1 small black coffee

TEA-TIME
Tea with lemon

DINNER
2-egg mushroom omelette. Serve with 1 tablespoon of broccoli and 2 grilled tomatoes.
1 fruit yoghurt
1 black coffee

BEFORE RETIRING
1 large glass of mineral water

Day 5
BREAKFAST
1 bowl of 6–8 stewed figs
1 black coffee

Four-Week Diets 109

MID-MORNING
1 glass of grapefruit juice or mineral water

LUNCH
1 slimmer's open sandwich made with 1 slice of wholemeal bread, a little butter, a small carton of cottage cheese, tomato, watercress, and 10–14 grapes

Plus 1 black coffee

TEA-TIME
Tea with lemon

DINNER
2 slices of grilled liver and 2 slices of bacon, served with grilled mushrooms, grilled tomatoes and a mixed green salad
1 crispbread
1 glass of apple juice
1 small black coffee

BEFORE RETIRING
1 glass of mineral water

Day 6
BREAKFAST
1 whole grapefruit, no sugar
1 crispbread with a little butter
1 black coffee

MID-MORNING
1 glass of apple juice or mineral water

LUNCH
2 oranges and 3 oz. (75 g) Edam or Cheddar cheese, chopped up and mixed together
1 fruit yoghurt
1 black coffee

TEA-TIME
Tea with lemon

DINNER
2 poached eggs on 3 tablespoons of cooked spinach
1 bowl of fresh fruit salad
1 small black coffee

BEFORE RETIRING
1 glass of mineral water

Day 7

BREAKFAST
1 carton of natural yoghurt, mixed with a little honey
1 small, sliced banana
1 cup of black coffee

MID-MORNING
1 glass of orange juice or mineral water

LUNCH
4 oz. (125 g) peeled shrimps with a wedge of lemon and a green salad
1 thin slice of wholemeal bread and a small piece of Edam or Cheddar cheese
1 black coffee

TEA-TIME
Tea with lemon

DINNER
3–4 slices of cold or hot roast lamb, no fat, served with 1 tomato and 1 tablespoon of broccoli
1 bowl of fresh fruit salad
1 glass of white wine

BEFORE RETIRING
1 glass of mineral water

The second, third and fourth weeks are the same as the first.

SLIMMER'S LUNCH PLAN DIET
(average weight loss 12 lb. in four weeks)

No matter how determined you may be to lose weight, there is no doubt that for people who take a packed lunch to work, this is the most testing time. Those who are lucky enough not to have to bother about their waistlines, can at least resort to meat pies, savoury flans, scotch eggs and fruit pies for some variety. But the majority of slimmers find it next to impossible to fit any of these into a diet, and still have some part of the daily calorie allowance left for the evening meal. The best many people can do to overcome the problem is to pack the eternal lettuce and tomato. That might do for just the odd day a month, but what about the rest of the time? Unless the packed lunch is appetising each day and contains plenty of variety, the slimmer is almost bound to think the effort not worthwhile and abandon the diet completely.

But with a little thought beforehand, packed mid-day meals can be the envy of the bread-roll brigade. Each of the ideas below provides approximately 350–400 calories. But do remember that if you are going to lose weight on this kind of diet, then it is important you start the day with a fairly well-balanced breakfast, restricting the kind of food you know to be fattening, and that your dinner is a sensible but light meal. If your calorie allowance is 1000 a day, it is likely that there will be room for only ½ pint (275 ml) of milk. If teas and coffees are taken black throughout the day, then most of this milk can be saved for breakfast and an evening drink. You might try spending a little extra on speciality teas which taste much better without milk and are served with a little lemon.

You will need a few containers of different sizes with your packed meals and a thermos flask. The most useful ones are shallow, square boxes, or tiny polythene containers shaped like moulds which can take liquid sauces, and round dish shapes, all with well-fitting lids. Hot stews will require a thermos flask with a wide neck.

Now all you need do is set aside a little time the evening before work, or find the will to get up two minutes earlier in the morning to prepare your mid-day meal.

(i) Consommé and cheese and vegetable medley: Use canned or home-made consommé, and pour into the thermos flask. Take a small box of crudités (raw vegetables) to eat with the soup. Slice into matchstick-size strips carrots, cucumber and celery. Cut radishes into roses. Take these to work in cold water so that they remain crisp.

(ii) Cheese and vegetable salad: Tear lettuce roughly, cube 2 oz. (50 g) of Edam cheese and as much cucumber as you like. Mix with 2 oz. (50g) of cooked and cooled broad beans. Season well and toss in 1 tablespoon of fresh French dressing. Finish the meal with 1 satsuma, or 1 small apple, and a glass of tomato juice.

(iii) Pear in walnut dressing: Place ½ a pear, either fresh or if canned, well drained, on a bed of lettuce in a square, polythene box. Surround with quartered tomatoes and diced cucumber. Make a dressing by mixing 2 tablespoons of low-calorie salad dressing with 1 oz. (25 g) of very finely grated Edam cheese and ½ oz. (15 g) of chopped walnuts.

Follow this with a salad of sliced orange and 6 grapes, and a syrup made from 1 teaspoon of sugar and a little water.

(iv) Prawn and cheese open sandwich: Cut a slice of wholemeal bread to fit the square box and spread with a thin layer of butter. Place in the box and top with successive layers of mustard and cress. Add about 1½ oz. (40 g) of grated Gouda cheese and 2 oz. (50 g) of prawns. Season well. Follow this with minted grapefruit. Segment 1 large grapefruit and place in a round container. Top with a little chopped mint.

(v) Cheesy chicken: Remove the skin from a 10 oz. (275 g) chicken joint, spread with Worcestershire sauce and then a little oil. Grill for about 15–20 minutes, turning occasionally. Place 1 oz. (25 g) of cheese on top of the joint, and grill until well brown. Allow to cool. Take a cold ratatouille made from sliced aubergines, courgettes, tomatoes and onions, all cooked in a pan with very little water. You may also have a soda water to drink, and some fresh orange slices to eat as a dessert.

Four-Week Diets 113

(vi) Eggs with curry dressing: Cook 1½ oz. (40 g) of rice in stock rather than water, drain and cool. Then hard-boil 1 egg, shell and cool. Place the rice and egg in a box and take curry dressing in a separate small container, plus 1 fresh orange juice. Prepare the curry dressing by adding as much curry paste to your liking and taste to 3 tablespoons of low-calorie salad dressing. Mix together, and you have a delicious curry paste. Plus you may have 1 small apple or satsuma.

(vii) Carbonnade of beef: This is a possibility if you have facilities at work to sit down to a hot meal with a plate, knife and fork. A wide neck flask is essential. Make the carbonnade from very lean stewing beef. Cook with sliced onions, tomato puree, and a little flour for thickening. Use equal quantities of ale and stock. One portion consists of 4 oz. (125 g) of beef and 5 oz. (150 g) of sauce. A salad of shredded, cooked red cabbage and onion goes well with this, and if a little vinegar or lemon plus herbs are added to the vegetables they will keep their red colour. You may also have a portion of raspberries and a fresh orange juice to drink.

(viii) Ham and asparagus roll: Cut 2 slices of wholemeal bread, remove the crust and flatten them with a rolling pin. Spread with a little butter, and place a small slice of lean ham and 1 asparagus spear on each, and then roll up. Follow with 1 oz. (25 g) of cheese and 2 crackers, and a grapefruit juice.

(ix) Apple and coleslaw starter: Remove the core from an eating apple. Scoop out a little of the flesh. Make a filling from finely grated white cabbage, plus 1 tablespoon of low-calorie salad dressing and ½ oz. (15 g) of raisins. Press the filling well down into the apple. Eat any remaining filling separately.

Follow with 2 oz. (50 g) of liver paté, and 2 starch-reduced crispbreads, plus a herbal tea and a natural yoghurt.

(x) Potted meat: Mix together 1½ oz. (40 g) of very lean, minced cooked beef or pork, ½ oz. (15 g) of butter, 1½ teaspoons of bottled fruit sauce (HP Sauce), salt and pepper, and pack into a mould (these quantities are sufficient for one portion). If pork is used, make salad of

1 diced apple tossed in lemon juice, chopped prunes and watercress. If beef, use shredded red cabbage, with chopped onions, and 1 tablespoon of low-calorie French dressing. Follow with citrus fruit salad and 1 glass of tomato juice.

(xi) Italian tuna: Cook 1 oz. (25 g) of wholewheat pasta rings, drain and cool. Skin and deseed 2 tomatoes and chop roughly. Mix these well with ½ a small onion, chopped, with a pinch of mixed herbs. Add the pasta rings and pack in a plastic container. Top with 3 oz. (75 g) of drained tuna fish and 1 oz. (25 g) of grated cheese. Follow with a glass of tomato juice to drink.

WEEKENDS ONLY DIET
(average weight loss 7–10 lb. in four weeks)

A weekend only diet, which can still enable you to lose up to 10 lb. in four weeks, providing that what you eat the rest of the week is sensible and not over-indulging.

BREAKFAST
½ melon (there are many varieties to choose from)
1 apple cut into quarters and each quarter spread with a little honey (eat together with melon)
1 glass of fruit juice

Plus 1 small cup of tea with lemon only

MID-MORNING
1 tangerine or 1 orange

LUNCH
Large glass of fresh orange juice or you can use tinned or frozen. To the juice add 1 banana either thinly sliced or mashed; then it's ready to drink.

TEA-TIME
1 tangerine or 1 orange

DINNER
1 whole grapefruit. Cut in half and remove segments. Chop segments up together with 4–5 black or white grapes and 2 teaspoons of chopped almonds. Return mixture to 'shells', spread with a teaspoon of runny honey on each and place under a hot grill for about 3–4 minutes.

Plus 1 small cup of tea with lemon (no milk, no sugar)

STRAWBERRY, BANANA AND YOGHURT DIET
(average weight loss 15–20 lb. in four weeks)

The main ingredients of this diet are fruit and yoghurt, an ideal diet in summertime. Good weight loss is achieved with an eating pattern of three days 'on', two days 'off'. On 'off' days eat a diet high in protein – fish, meat, eggs – plus lots of green salads and fresh fruit.

FIRST MEAL
1 glass of milk
1 banana
1 fruit flavoured yoghurt

SECOND MEAL
4 oz. (125 g) of strawberries or raspberries
1 plain yoghurt
1 cup of black coffee

THIRD MEAL
1 banana
1 plain yoghurt
1 cup of black coffee

FOURTH MEAL
Make a fruit salad with 1 banana and 2 oz. (50 g) strawberries or raspberries
1 yoghurt
1 glass of lemonade, made from the juice of 1 fresh lemon, topped up with soda water or ordinary water, and 1 teaspoon of sugar

FIFTH MEAL
1 banana
1 fruit yoghurt
1 cup of black coffee

SIXTH MEAL
1 banana or 2 oz. (50 g) of strawberries or raspberries

SEVENTH MEAL
1 plain yoghurt

EIGHTH MEAL
1 banana
4 oz. (125 g) of strawberries or raspberries
1 glass of milk
1 thin slice of wholemeal bread with a little butter, and spread with 1 teaspoon of honey

Coffee can be sweetened with artificial sweeteners, and fruit with the juice of a fresh orange. Sugar is only permitted once during the day in the lemonade.

INCENTIVE DIET
(average weight loss 12–15 lb. in four weeks)

Here is a four-week diet plan which should enable you to lose 12–15 lb. The first day is a fasting day, so plan to start the diet on a non-working day. The first day will naturally show weight loss which is a great incentive to a weak-willed slimmer.

Day 1 (a fasting day)
Drink up to 8 glasses of mineral water throughout the day and up to ¾ lb. (425 g) grapes *or* two grapefruits, peeled and segmented

Day 2
BREAKFAST
Either 1 whole grapefruit without sugar *or* 8 prunes
1 small cup of mint, rosehip or camomile tea
1 small carton of natural yoghurt mixed with 1 tablespoon of wheatgerm and 1 tablespoon of natural bran
1 glass of mineral water

LUNCH
A 2-egg omelette cooked in a non-stick pan and served with a salad made from fresh raw bean sprouts, chopped spring onions, and a little grated cheese or walnuts over the top. Add a salad dressing made with oil and cider vinegar.

Plus 1 glass of mineral water

TEA-TIME
1 glass of mineral water or 1 cup of herbal tea

DINNER
4–5 good slices of breast of chicken, no skin, served with 2 green vegetables, steamed
1 slice of natural wholemeal bread, with a thin slice of Cheddar cheese
1 glass of mineral water or 1 cup of herbal tea

Four-Week Diets

Day 3
BREAKFAST
The same as for Day 2

MID-MORNING
1 glass of mineral water or 1 cup of herbal tea

LUNCH
1 large helping, about 6 tablespoons, of fresh fruit salad
2 oz. (50 g) of Cheddar cheese, cubed
1 glass of mineral water or herbal tea

TEA-TIME
1 glass of mineral water or 1 cup of herbal tea

DINNER
1 bowl of fresh vegetable soup, made with soup cubes, or consommé
1 medium-sized jacket potato. Remove the insides from the jacket and mash with 4 oz. (125 g) of grated cheese and 2 chopped spring onions. Return to potato skin. Serve with a good-sized mixed salad, and a dressing of cider vinegar and oil.

Plus 1 glass of mineral water or herbal tea

Day 4
BREAKFAST
The same as for Day 2

MID-MORNING
1 glass of mineral water or 1 cup of herbal tea

LUNCH
2 tablespoons brown rice, served with stir-fry vegetables of your choice, cooked Chinese-style in a small amount of oil. Cook vegetables quickly.
1 pear, apple *or* ½ grapefruit

TEA-TIME
1 glass of mineral water or 1 cup of herbal tea

DINNER
½ grapefruit
1 poached egg
1 thin slice of natural wholemeal bread with Cheddar cheese

Day 5
BREAKFAST
The same as for Day 2

MID-MORNING
1 glass of mineral water or 1 cup of herbal tea

LUNCH
1 slice of wholemeal bread, spread thinly with butter, and topped with 2 oz. (50 g) of Edam cheese. Serve with a tomato, onion and cucumber salad.

Plus 1 glass of mineral water or herbal tea

TEA-TIME
1 glass of mineral water or 1 cup of herbal tea

DINNER
4 oz. (125 g) cold cooked sea food, such as shrimps, crab, lobster or flaked haddock. Serve with celery, mushroom, tomato, and spring onion salad, dressed with oil and cider vinegar.

Plus either 1 fresh apple, *or* pear, *or* peach *or* ½ grapefruit
1 glass of mineral water or herbal tea

Day 6
BREAKFAST
The same as for Day 2

MID-MORNING
1 glass of mineral water or 1 cup of herbal tea

LUNCH
6 oz. (175 g) grilled steak, veal, or lean lamb. Serve with a green salad.
½ grapefruit
1 glass of mineral water or herbal tea

TEA-TIME
1 glass of mineral water or 1 cup of herbal tea

DINNER
Grill 2 slices of back bacon really dry. Pat with a paper towel to remove any excess fat. Crumble over 2 handfuls of freshly washed raw spinach, chopped and dressed with a little oil and lemon.

Plus 1 slice of wholemeal bread, topped with Cheddar cheese
1 glass of mineral water or herbal tea

Day 7
BREAKFAST
The same as for Day 2

MID-MORNING
1 glass of mineral water or 1 cup of herbal tea

LUNCH
Mix a large salad with a dressing of oil and lemon juice. Add 1 chopped hard boiled egg and 2 slices of pineapple.

Plus 1 glass of mineral water or 1 cup of herbal tea

TEA-TIME
1 glass of mineral water or 1 cup of herbal tea

DINNER
1 portion of grilled sole or any other white fish served with lemon and a raw mushroom salad with a little yoghurt dressing
1 slice of wholemeal bread, with a thin slice of Edam cheese
1 glass of mineral water or 1 cup of herbal tea

Repeat the diet for a further three weeks; always make certain that the first day is a non-working day.

Two-Month Diets

These diets should be treated as a complete re-education of bad eating habits, and as a start to a whole new way of life that will hopefully remain permanent.

TOWN AND COUNTRY DIET
(average weight loss 28–30 lb. in two months)

This high-protein reducing diet provides for a daily allowance of approximately 1200 calories, and over 100 grams of protein, an unusual amount for a diet with so few calories. Carbohydrates are reduced to a minimum. Here are some important rules to follow on the Town and Country Diet:

1. Eat lean meat, trim off all visible fat. Meat should be boiled, grilled, or roasted, never fried.
2. Four portions of vegetables should be eaten daily. One of them should be high in vitamin A. Eat fresh or stewed fruit without sugar.
3. A saccharine sweetener or a sugar substitute may be used to sweeten food.
4. You may have salt, pepper, spices, herbs, herb essences, vinegar, tea, black coffee, lemon juice, gelatine, Marmite or Bovril, in moderate amounts.
5. Avoid carbohydrates (i.e. starches and sugars). These are in ordinary bread and crispbreads, other than those mentioned in the diet sheet; flour and all foods made with it, such as puddings, cakes, biscuits, pastries, spaghetti, macaroni etc.; thickened soups and sauces, including packet soups and thickened tinned soups; breakfast cereals and other cereals, such as rice, cornflour etc.; potatoes, parsnips, beetroot, peas, haricot and baked beans, lentils and others; sugar, jams and jams sweetened with sorbitol, syrups, sweets, chocolates, including diabetic chocolate, cocoa, malted milk products, cream and ice-cream, fruit tinned in sugar, or sorbitol, dried fruit, nuts, cordials and other sweetened fruit juices; oils and fats other than the amount stated on the diet sheet; fish tinned in oil; mayonnaise, salad dressing and chutney; sausages, beer, stout and alcoholic drinks.
6. Milk is the most important individual food and you are allowed ½ pint (275 ml) of skimmed milk a day. You are also allowed each day up to 3 oz. (75 g) of butter plus 4 starch-reduced crispbreads, and it is important that you do not go over this allowance.
7. When stated, eat only from the groups of foods listed at the end of the diet.

This diet should be looked upon as a total re-education of your eating habits and one in which the whole family can join you. *You* choose the kinds of foods you want to eat from the lists given, and this reduces the temptation of selecting the wrong kinds of food. Eat only from the foods listed and you and your family can enjoy a more healthy and rewarding way of life. For growing children you can modify the diet and include each day at least half a pint of milk (275 ml) and up to three slices of wholemeal bread.

BREAKFAST
1 serving of fruit high in vitamin C content such as those in Group A
1 egg or a small serving of other protein food from Group B
1 crispbread with a little butter
1 cup of coffee or tea with milk

MID-MORNING
1 cup of tea or coffee with milk or 1 cup of Marmite

LUNCH
1 cup of low-calorie soup from Group C
Lean meat or other protein food from Group D. Serve with a portion of vegetables from Group E.
1 serving of salad from Group F, but no salad oil or sugar
1 crispbread with a little butter
Milk from the allowance made into an egg custard or milk jelly, or substituted by fat-free yoghurt
2 servings of fruit from Group A
1 cup of coffee or tea with milk

TEA-TIME
1 crispbread with butter
Marmite or Bovril, if desired
1 cup of tea with milk

DINNER
1 cup of low-calorie soup from Group C
Lean meat or other protein food from Group D
1 serving of low-calorie cooked vegetables from Group E
1 serving of salad from Group F without salad oil or sugar
1 starch-reduced crispbread with butter
Milk from the allowance, made into an egg custard or

milk jelly or substituted by fat-free yoghurt
2 servings of fruit from Group A
1 cup of tea or coffee with milk

BEFORE RETIRING
1 cup of Marmite, tea or the remainder of milk from the allowance

GROUP A – FRUITS, UNSWEETENED
apple, 1 small, baked or stewed, 3 oz. (75g)
apricots, canned including liquid, 5 oz. (150g)
banana, 1 small, 1½ oz. (40 g)
blackberries, fresh, 4 oz. (125 g)
cantaloup melon*, 3½ oz. (90 g)
cherries, canned including liquid, 5 oz. (150 g)
grapefruit*, 3½ oz. (90 g)
grapefruit juice*, 3½ oz. (90 g)
honeydew melon, 3½ oz. (90 g)
orange*, 1 small, 2½ oz. (65 g)
orange juice*, 2 oz. (50 g)
peach, fresh, 1 medium large, 3 oz. (75 g)
peaches, canned including liquid, 5 oz. (150 g)
pear, fresh, 1 medium, 2½ oz. (65 g)
pears, canned including liquid, 5 oz. (150 g)
pineapple, fresh, 2 oz. (50 g)
pineapple, canned including liquid, 5 oz. (150 g)
plums, fresh, 3 oz. (75 g)
plums, canned including liquid, 5 oz. (150 g)
raspberries, fresh or canned including liquid, 5 oz. (150 g)
strawberries*, 3 oz. (75 g)
watermelon, 4 oz. (125 g)

*These fruits are rich in Vitamin C, and at least 1 serving should be taken each day.

GROUP B – HIGH PROTEIN FOODS FOR BREAKFAST
bacon, lean, crisp, grilled and drained dry, 1 oz. (25 g)
cheese, Cheddar, ¾ oz. (20 g)
cheese, cottage, 2 oz. (50 g)
cheese, Edam, 1 oz. (25 g)
cheese, Gouda, 2 oz. (50 g)
cheese, Swiss, ¾ oz. (20 g)
egg, poached, boiled or scrambled, with 1 oz. (25 g) butter and milk from the allowance

Two-Month Diets 127

GROUP C – SOUPS, LOW CALORIE
beef broth, 5 oz. (150 g)
beef broth with vegetables, 5 oz. (150 g)
bouillon or consommé, 5 oz. (150 g)
onion soup, clear, 5 oz. (150 g)
tomato soup, clear, 5 oz. (150 g)
tomato juice, as an alternative to soup, 4 oz. (125 g)
vegetable broth, 5 oz. (150 g)

GROUP D – MEAT, FISH AND OTHER PROTEIN FOODS
beef, lean, roast, or corned beef, 3½ oz. (90 g)
beef, lean, silverside, 3½ oz. (90 g)
chicken, roast, 5 oz. (150 g)
cod steak, 7 oz. (200 g)
grouse, roast, 6 oz. (175 g)
haddock, 6 oz. (175 g)
halibut steak, 6 oz. (175 g)
ham, lean, boiled, 3½ oz. (90 g)
hare, weighed with bones and stewed without flour, 8 oz. (225 g)
kidney, stewed without flour, 5 oz. (150 g)
lamb, lean leg of, or shoulder roasted, 3½ oz. (90 g)
liver, grilled, 5 oz. (150 g)
lobster, mackerel, salmon or shrimps, 5 oz. (150 g)
ox tongue, lean, pickled, 3½ oz. (90 g)
oysters without shells, 8 oz. (225 g)
partridge, roast, 4½ oz. (140 g)
rabbit, weighed with bones and stewed without flour, 8 oz. (225 g)
salmon, canned, 4 oz. (125 g)
sole, 7 oz. (200 g)
sweetbread, stewed without flour, 4 oz. (125 g)
tripe, stewed without flour, 6 oz. (175 g)
turkey, roast, 5 oz. (150 g)
veal, leg, or shoulder roasted, 3½ oz. (90 g)
venison, roast, 5 oz. (150 g)

GROUP E – VEGETABLES, LOW CALORIE
artichokes, globe, 5 oz. (150 g)
asparagus, 3 oz. (75 g)
beans, French or runner, 5 oz. (150 g)
broccoli*, 2½ oz. (65 g)
Brussels sprouts, 2 oz. (50 g)
cabbage*, 3 oz. (75 g)

carrots*, 2 oz. (50 g)
cauliflower, 3 oz. (75 g)
kale cabbage*, 1 oz. (25 g)
leeks, 1½ oz. (40 g)
marrow, 5 oz. (150 g)
mushrooms, 5 oz. (150 g)
onions, 2½ oz. (65 g)
peas, green, 1 oz. (25 g)
sauerkraut, 2 oz. (50 g)
sea kale, 5 oz. (150 g)
spinach*, 2 oz. (50 g)
spring greens, 3 oz. (75 g)
swedes, 2 oz. (50 g)
tomatoes, canned, 2 oz. (50 g)
tomato juice, canned, 2 oz. (50 g)
turnips, white, 3 oz. (75 g)

GROUP F – VEGETABLES, RAW, FOR SALADS
cabbage, white, 1½ oz. (40 g)
cabbage, red, 2 oz. (50 g)
carrots*, 2 oz. (50 g)
celery stalks, 3 oz. (75 g)
chicory, 3 oz. (75 g)
cress*, mustard and cress, 3 oz. (75 g)
cress*, watercress, 2½ oz. (65 g)
cucumber, 3 oz. (75 g)
endive*, 3 oz. (75 g)
lettuce*, 5 small leaves, 3 oz. (75 g)
pepper, green, 1½ oz. (40 g)
pimento*, 1 small, 1 oz. (25 g)
radishes, red, 2½ oz. (65 g)
spring onions, 1 oz. (25 g)
tomatoes*, 2½ oz. (65 g)

*These vegetables are rich in Vitamin A. At least 1 serving should be taken each day.

TOTAL DIET
(average weight loss 28–30 lb. in two months)

Note that on this diet lunches are a light meal. You are allowed up to 5 teacups of liquid each day – it can be either tea with lemon, black coffee or mineral/spring water. Sugar is not permitted, but you may use artificial sweetener.

Day 1
BREAKFAST
½ a grapefruit, no sugar
1 cup of tea with lemon or 1 glass of fruit juice

LUNCH
1 mixed salad using all kinds of fresh vegetables served with a little oil and lemon only

DINNER
1 portion of steamed fish, served with steamed carrots and Brussels sprouts
1 baked apple

Day 2
BREAKFAST
1 glass of fresh fruit juice
1 apple
1 cup of lemon tea

LUNCH
1 carton of yoghurt and 1 piece of fruit

DINNER
1 small, mixed salad with 1 small baked potato and a little margarine
1 bowl of stewed apple

Day 3
BREAKFAST
1 glass of fresh fruit juice
1 slice of wholemeal bread, toasted, and spread with margarine
1 cup of lemon tea

LUNCH
1 mixed salad using all kinds of fresh vegetables served with a little oil and lemon only

DINNER
1 portion of lamb, served with broccoli and a side salad of tomatoes, pickled red cabbage and cucumber
1 bowl of fruit salad

Day 4
BREAKFAST
1 bowl of muesli with yoghurt
1 glass of fresh fruit juice or lemon tea

LUNCH
1 bowl of vegetable soup
1 dry cracker

DINNER
1 vegetable omelette with 1 baked potato and a little margarine
½ a melon or a few grapes

Day 5
BREAKFAST
1 glass of fresh fruit juice
½ a grapefruit without sugar
1 cup of black coffee, without sugar

LUNCH
1 mixed salad

DINNER
1 portion of steamed fish, served with peas and celery
½ a melon

Day 6
BREAKFAST
1 cup of lemon tea
½ a grapefruit

LUNCH
1 average-sized grilled steak and a mixed salad

DINNER
Cheese salad, with 1 small baked potato and a little margarine
1 bowl of fruit salad

Day 7
BREAKFAST
1 slice of wholemeal bread, toasted, spread with margarine
1 boiled or scrambled egg
1 cup of black coffee, no sugar

LUNCH
1 portion of chicken with peas and carrots and 1 small baked potato

DINNER
1 bowl of fresh fruit and yoghurt or a mixed salad

MISS GREAT BRITAIN DIET
(average weight loss 28–30 lb. in two months)

I originally designed this diet for a Miss Great Britain. Now I am not suggesting that you would all like to look like a Miss Great Britain, but if you do need to lose weight why not try the diet?

Day 1
ON RISING
1 glass of hot water, to which is added a slice of orange

BREAKFAST
2 tablespoons of bran, eaten dry. This is to prevent constipation, and to help if you already suffer from it.
1 small carton of natural yoghurt
1 piece of fresh fruit, but not bananas
1 small cup of tea without milk or sugar. Try the herbal or mint teas, since they are more refreshing.

LUNCH
1 boiled egg
1 crispbread plus margarine
10–12 grapes
1 glass of mineral water

DINNER
4 tablespoons fresh fruit salad
1 thin slice of wholemeal bread with margarine
2 oz. (50 g) Edam, Gouda or Cheddar cheese
1 glass of mineral water

Day 2
BREAKFAST
Exactly the same as Day 1

LUNCH
1 small carton of cottage cheese
2 thin slices of corned beef
1 pickled cucumber
1 crispbread with margarine
1 glass of mineral water

DINNER
4 oz. (125 g) peeled shrimps
A salad, made with sliced green and red pepper, celery and lettuce, and dressed with lemon juice and black pepper
1 thin slice of wholemeal bread with margarine
1 pear
1 glass of mineral water

Day 3
BREAKFAST
Exactly the same as Day 1

LUNCH
3 tablespoons grated Edam, Gouda or Cheddar cheese. Pile on top of 2 crispbreads, and top with thin slices of apple and onion
1 fruit yoghurt
1 glass of mineral water

DINNER
2-egg omelette stuffed with mushrooms. Cook, if possible, in a non-stick pan, or use a little margarine.
1 glass of mineral water

Day 4
BREAKFAST
Exactly the same as Day 1

LUNCH
4–5 slices of cold chicken, without the skin. Serve on a bed of sliced lettuce, tomato, cucumber and onion.
1 apple
1 glass of mineral water

DINNER
3 tablespoons cooked fresh spinach, on which is served 1 poached egg
1 thin slice of wholemeal bread with margarine
1 glass of mineral water

Day 5
BREAKFAST
Exactly the same as Day 1

LUNCH
A large plate of mixed salad, using any vegetables you like, and dressed with a little oil and lemon
1 crispbread with margarine
1 fresh peach or 10–12 grapes
1 glass of mineral water

DINNER
2 medium fillets of grilled white fish. Serve with 2 or 3 grilled tomatoes and 2 grilled courgettes, with a wedge of lemon.
1 glass of mineral water

Day 6
BREAKFAST
Exactly the same as Day 1

LUNCH
3 tablespoons fresh fruit salad, served with 1 small carton of cottage cheese
1 thin slice of wholemeal bread with margarine
1 glass of mineral water

DINNER
2 medium slices of grilled liver or 2 lean lamb cutlets
1 tablespoon each of runner beans and carrots
1 glass of mineral water

Day 7 (a fast day)
You are allowed to drink up to 6 glasses of mineral water and eat 2 oranges throughout the day. Peel and quarter the oranges, leave them in the fridge, and whenever you feel hungry, have a couple of orange quarters and a glass of water. It will then seem as if you are eating and drinking at least something regularly throughout the day.

'I LOVE TO EAT' DIET
(average weight loss 20–25 lb. in two months)

This is a super diet for those people who love eating. Although it is balanced to ensure a safe 1,200 calories a day, it is also full of healthgiving foods that will not only aid weight loss, but hair, skin and general appearance will also benefit.

1. Each day, choose 1 of the 7 breakfasts, 7 light meals and 7 main meals that are set out below, plus any vegetables from your vegetables nibble bowl, and 1 of the special nibble treats.

2. You are allowed 1 pint (575 ml) of milk each day for use in tea and coffee, and where mentioned in recipes (it might be a good idea to separate your own bottle of milk from the family's supply).

3. There is no need to limit the intake of low-calorie liquids such as water, meat extract drinks, etc. Tea and coffee are also unlimited, as long as you only use milk from the allowance and artificial sweeteners.

4. A list of fruits for the fruit portions mentioned is given at the end, along with a list of allowable nibbles and recipes for some of the delicious dishes.

BREAKFASTS
Choose *one* of the following:

(i) ½ a grapefruit, no sugar
1 boiled egg
1 thin slice of wholemeal toast, lightly buttered
1 cup of tea or coffee with milk from the allowance

(ii) 1 small glass of fresh orange juice
2 rashers of streaky bacon, well grilled, with 1 sliced tomato
1 thin slice of unbuttered wholemeal toast
1 cup of tea or coffee

(iii) 1 small glass of tomato juice
1 rasher of back bacon, fried, with 2 oz. (50 g) mushrooms
1 thin slice of lightly buttered wholemeal toast.
1 cup of tea or coffee

(iv) 1 portion of fresh fruit, see at the end of the list
2 oz. (50 g) grilled kidneys with 2 oz. (50 g) mushrooms, cooked in their own juices
1 starch-reduced crispbread, no butter
1 cup of tea or coffee

(v) 1 oz. (25 g) breakfast cereal, with milk from the allowance
Creamed mushrooms made as follows:
Cook 4 oz. (125 g) mushrooms in their own juices. Remove from the heat, and stir in ½ a carton of natural yoghurt, salt, pepper and a dash of Worcestershire sauce, and then serve on 1 thin slice of wholemeal toast.

Plus 1 cup of tea or coffee

(vi) Breakfast pizza, made as follows:
Toast 1 thin slice of wholemeal bread. Then cover with 1 oz. (25 g) sliced mushrooms, 1 slice of tomato and 1 oz. (25 g) thinly sliced Edam cheese. Place under a hot grill until the cheese begins to melt. Garnish with 1 black olive or 1 pickled walnut.

Plus 1 piece of fresh fruit
1 cup of tea or coffee

(vii) ½ a grapefruit, no sugar
1 scrambled egg with 2 tablespoons of milk from the allowance
1 thin slice of wholemeal toast, lightly buttered
1 cup of tea or coffee

LIGHT MEALS
(i) Savoury baked eggs, made as follows:
Mix together 2 oz. (50 g) of mushrooms, sliced, 2 tablespoons of evaporated milk, salt and pepper. Put in a small oven-proof dish. Break an egg on top and sprinkle with ½ oz. (15 g) of grated Edam cheese. Bake at 350°F/180°C or Gas Mark 4 for approximately 15 minutes, until the egg is firm and the cheese has melted. Serve with a mixed green salad.

Plus 2 rye crispbreads, very lightly buttered
1 small glass of tomato juice

(ii) Tomato cauliflower cheese, made as follows:
Cover a large portion of boiled cauliflower with tomato sauce, prepared from 5 tablespoons of cream of tomato soup and a dash of Worcestershire sauce. Sprinkle over the top 1 oz. (25 g) of grated Edam cheese. Heat under a hot grill until the cheese melts.

Plus 1 unbuttered rye crispbread
1 portion of fresh fruit

(iii) Mushroom omelette, made with ½ oz. (15 g) of butter, 2 eggs, 2 oz. (50 g) mushrooms, and watercress
1 cup of tea or coffee, no sugar, or meat extract

(iv) Toasted cheese pineapple sandwich, made as follows:
Toast 2 thin slices of wholemeal bread on one side only. Mix together 1 oz. (25 g) of grated Edam cheese and 1 tablespoon of drained, crushed pineapple, and sandwich between toasted sides of bread. Toast on the outside and serve hot with watercress.

Plus 1 portion of fresh fruit

(v) Cheese coleslaw, made as follows:
Prepare a dressing from 1 tablespoon of natural yoghurt, a little vinegar, pinch of salt, pepper and sugar. Mix together 2 oz. (50 g) of shredded white cabbage, ½ a small red eating apple, cored and diced, and toss in 2 teaspoons of lemon juice, 1 tablespoon of grated onion, 2 oz. (50 g) of diced Edam cheese. Add the dressing and toss well together. Serve garnished with parsley or chicory or watercress.

Plus 1 portion of fresh fruit

(vi) Mushroom and ham cocotte, made as follows:
Beat together 1 egg, 4 tablespoons of milk from the allowance, salt and pepper to taste. Stir in 1 oz. (25 g) of sliced mushrooms, 1 oz. (25 g) of chopped lean ham, 1 teaspoon of freshly chopped parsley. Pour into a lightly greased individual ovenproof dish, and bake at 325°F/160°C or Gas Mark 3 for 20 minutes until set. Garnish with fresh parsley and serve with green salad vegetables, and 1 small slice of lightly buttered wholemeal bread.

Plus 1 portion of fresh fruit

(vii) Sardines au gratin, made as follows:
Toast 1 slice of wholemeal bread on 1 side. Place 2 sardines in tomato sauce on the untoasted side. Sprinkle with lemon juice, a little grated onion and a little chopped parsley. Cover with 1 oz. (25 g) of grated Edam cheese and melt under a hot grill. Serve hot.

Plus 1 portion of fresh fruit

MAIN MEALS
Choose *one* of the following (the asterisks indicate that the recipe is given at the end of the diet):

(i) 1 portion of mushroom and Edam cheese roast, with tomato sauce.* Serve with a mixed salad made from lettuce, chicory, cucumber, watercress, pepper and tomatoes, no dressing.

Plus 6 oz. (175 g) portion of yellow melon, no sugar

(ii) Liver casserole, made with 6 oz. (175 g) lamb's liver, 2 oz. (50 g) sliced onions, 2 oz. (50 g) sliced mushrooms and 4 oz. (125 g) canned tomatoes. Add a pinch of mixed herbs and seasoning. Serve with 4 oz. (125 g) boiled celery, 3 oz. (75 g) brussels sprouts, or other leafy green vegetables.

Plus 1 oz. (25 g) Edam cheese
1 rye crispbread

(iii) Baked chicken joint with mushrooms, made by wrapping in foil a chicken joint, 9 oz. (250 g) in weight, and 2 oz. (50 g) of button mushrooms, all of which have been sprinkled with lemon juice, salt and pepper. Bake for 40 minutes at 375°F/190°C or Gas Mark 5. Serve with 3 oz. (75 g) carrots and 4 oz. (125 g) broccoli or any other leafy green vegetables.

Plus 1 oz. (25 g) Edam cheese
2 crackers

(iv) 1 portion of cheesy yoghurt topped fish.* Serve with 2 oven-baked tomatoes and 4 oz. (125 g) of green beans.
1 portion of fresh fruit

(v) 1 portion of courgette or marrow Neapolitan.* Serve

with 1 rasher of well grilled bacon.
1 portion of fresh fruit

(vi) 1 portion of minced beef and aubergine fiesta.* Serve with a mixed green salad, no dressing.
2 oz. (50 g) vanilla ice-cream or a medium-sized banana

(vii) 1 portion of patio salad*
1 portion of fresh fruit

FRESH FRUIT PORTIONS:
1 medium-sized eating apple
1 small orange
4 oz. (125 g) fresh whole peaches
6 oz. (175 g) fresh whole apricots
4 oz. (125 g) fresh whole cherries
4 oz. (125 g) dessert gooseberries
6 oz. (175 g) grapefruit, peeled
1 medium-sized pear
3 oz. (75 g) fresh pineapple
6 oz. (175 g) raspberries
6 oz. (175 g) strawberries
1 tangerine, peeled

ALLOWABLE NIBBLES:
Vegetable nibble bowl This is to eat in between meals, when the hunger pangs strike. Store in the refrigerator a bowl of the following vegetables, sliced:
    cucumber
    tomatoes
    celery
    whole radishes
    button mushrooms
    rings of green pepper
    carrot sticks

Nibble treats Choose *one* only of these each day, either at the time of day when you reach your lowest ebb, or at the end of the day:
1 small bar of Milky Way
1 oz. (25 g) wine gums
1 oz. (25 g) fruit gums
1 oz. (25 g) liquorice allsorts

12 Twiglets
4 Cheddar cheese squares
3 Tuck biscuits
3 Energen cheese crispbreads
3 Nice biscuits
3 tea finger biscuits
3 Marie biscuits
1 chocolate wholemeal biscuit
¼ pint (150 ml) thick soup
1 carton natural yoghurt
1 small wine glass of medium sherry
1 measure of gin or whisky, with slim line tonic or bitter lemon or ginger ale

MAIN MEAL RECIPES
Mushroom and Edam Cheese Roast (serves 4)
1 large onion, peeled and chopped
1 large green pepper, deseeded and chopped
1 oz. (25 g) butter
4 oz. (125 g) mushrooms
4 oz. (125 g) brown breadcrumbs
3 eggs
seasoning
6 oz. (175 g) grated Edam cheese
a pinch of mixed herbs

Method
Gently fry onion and green pepper in the butter until soft, but not brown. Add sliced mushrooms, and cook for a further 2 minutes. Remove from heat and add the remaining ingredients, except the cheese and mixed herbs. Mix thoroughly. Then grease a 2 lb. (900 g) loaf tin and press the mixture into it. Sprinkle over with grated cheese and mixed herbs, and bake on the middle shelf of the oven at 350°F/180°C or Gas Mark 4 for 45 minutes. Serve hot with tomato sauce.

Tomato Sauce (serves 4)
Place in a liquidiser, or finely chop together a 15 oz. (425 g) can tomatoes, ½ a small onion, salt and pepper to taste and a dash of Worcestershire sauce. Heat in a pan for 5 minutes before serving.

Cheesy Yoghurt Topped Fish (serves 4)
1½ lb. (700 g) fresh or frozen cod or haddock fillets
2 × 5 oz. (150 g) cartons of natural low fat yoghurt
1 level teaspoon dry mustard
freshly ground pepper
6 oz. (175 g) grated Edam cheese
parsley to garnish

Method
Place fish in a lightly greased shallow baking dish. Mix together the yoghurt, mustard, pepper and 4 oz. (125 g) of cheese. Spread over the fish. Bake at 350°F/180°C or Gas Mark 4 for 25 minutes. Sprinkle with the remaining grated cheese. Replace in the oven for about 10 minutes or until cheese melts, and then garnish with sprigs of fresh parsley.

Courgette (or Marrow) Neapolitan (serves 4)
1 lb. (450 g) fresh tomatoes, skinned, or 15 oz. (425 g) can tomatoes
1 small onion, peeled and chopped
salt and pepper
1½ lb. (675 g) courgettes *or* 2 lb. (900 g) marrow
1 tablespoon flour
1 oz. (25 g) butter
8 oz. (225 g) Edam cheese, thinly sliced

Method
Chop up the tomatoes and heat in a saucepan with the onion, salt and pepper to taste, for 10 minutes, to make a thick tomato sauce. Slice the courgettes or marrow into ½" rings and then into quarters. Shake in a bag with flour to coat evenly. Melt the butter in a large frying pan, and fry the courgettes or marrow until brown on both sides. Put alternating layers of courgettes or marrow, the tomato mixture and the cheese in a shallow baking dish. Finish off with a layer of cheese. Bake on the top shelf of the oven at 375°F/190°C or Gas Mark 5 for 30 minutes. Serve topped with 1 rasher of well grilled bacon per serving.

Minced Beef and Aubergine Fiesta (serves 4)
1 lb. (450 g) lean minced beef
1 large onion, chopped
1 lb. (450 g) aubergines
boiling water

15 oz. (425 g) can tomatoes, drained
8 oz. (225 g) mushrooms, sliced
1 clove of garlic, peeled and crushed
¼ level teaspoon salt
freshly ground black pepper
4 oz. (125 g) Edam cheese, grated
chopped parsley for garnishing

Method

Fry the minced beef in a pan in its own fat until brown. Remove from pan with a slotted spoon, leaving the fat behind. Fry the onion in the fat until soft, but not brown. Add to the minced beef with salt and pepper to taste. Place the beef mixture in a lightly greased ovenproof dish. Then peel the aubergines, cut into 1" slices, and cut each slice into 4 triangular pieces. Put in a saucepan, cover with boiling water and boil for 10 minutes. Drain well. Roughly chop the tomatoes and mix with the aubergines, sliced mushrooms, garlic and seasoning. Spread over the minced beef. Bake uncovered towards the top of the oven at 400°F/200°C or Gas Mark 6 for about 20 minutes. Sprinkle with the grated cheese and bake for a further 10 minutes until the cheese has melted. Garnish with chopped parsley.

Patio Salad (serves 4)
a pinch of salt, pepper and sugar
⅛ level teaspoon dry mustard
1 dessertspoon vinegar
1 tablespoon salad oil
2 oz. (50 g) Edam cheese, diced
2 oz. (50 g) button mushrooms, cut into quarters
1 large stick of celery, diced
1 oz. (25 g) black olives
1 lettuce

Method

Prepare the dressing by shaking together the seasoning, mustard, vinegar and oil. Place all the other ingredients except the lettuce in a bowl. Pour over the dressing and mix well. Leave to stand for at least ½ an hour in a cold place. Serve on a bed of lettuce.

LEARN HOW TO OVERCOME TENSION AND STRESS IN ONLY 30 MINUTES A DAY!

The 10 day Relaxation Plan

DR ERIC TRIMMER

Stress is one of today's biggest killers. The pressures of modern living ensure that most of us at some time will suffer from anxiety and tension, becoming potential victims of stress-related disease. Dr Eric Trimmer explains how we can recognise the first symptoms of stress in our bodies, together with the factors which trigger them – and train ourselves to relax, without recourse to pills or alcohol.

* This is the first book to draw together a variety of disciplines, including yoga and autogenics, to produce a unique plan of simple exercises.
* The exercises are clearly illustrated and arranged in three programmes to suit all ages and levels of fitness.
* Just select the programme which suits you best – whether you're a housewife, pensioner or businessman – and in 10 days learn how to overcome tension and enjoy a healthy body and mind!

HEALTH AND FITNESS   0 7221 8605 3   £1.95

KITTY CAMPION'S
HANDBOOK OF HERBAL HEALTH

The natural way to a healthier life

Herbalism is the most natural way to get healthy and stay healthy. This detailed handbook written by a medical herbalist, tells you everything you need to know about herbs: how to identify them, collect them, cook with them and how to prepare traditional herbal remedies for headaches, high blood pressure, toothache, sunburn and many other common ailments. There's also advice on how to make refreshing herbal drinks and details of a complete herbal cleansing programme that will revitalise your body.

Covering hundreds of herbs and cures, KITTY CAMPION'S HANDBOOK OF HERBAL HEALTH will show you that herbal remedies are as effective today as they've always been. When you realise the natural alternatives, you may never have to take an aspirin again.

HEALTH AND MEDICINE   0 7221 2352 3   £2.95

JUDITH SAXTON

Bestselling author of *The Pride*

SOPHIE

She could hardly believe it was happening . . .

Especially when she looked back. Here was Sophie now – with a London flat, a good job at the television studios, and the kind of figure that was beginning to get her noticed. And particularly by Stephen, one of the TV directors.

A far cry from the Sophie of recent times – the fat girl from the provinces, the perennial party wallflower, who could only make friends with people as lonely as herself.

Had she consulted a fortune teller, she would have seen a bright future ahead of her. But would it lead in quite the direction she wanted? And, at the end of the road, would she recognise the girl in the crystal ball as herself?

GENERAL FICTION 0 7221 8646 0   £1.95

A selection of bestsellers from SPHERE

FICTION

HUSBANDS AND LOVERS	Ruth Harris	£2.95 ☐
SWITCH	William Bayer	£2.50 ☐
VITAL SIGNS	Barbara Wood	£2.95 ☐
THE ZURICH NUMBERS	Bill Granger	£2.75 ☐

FILM & TV TIE-INS

BOON	Anthony Masters	£2.50 ☐
LADY JANE	Anthony Smith	£1.95 ☐

NON-FICTION

LET'S FACE IT	Christine Piff	£2.50 ☐
A QUIET YEAR	Derek Tangye	£2.50 ☐
THE 1986 FAMILY WELCOME GUIDE	Jill Foster & Malcolm Hamer	£4.95 ☐
THE ABSOLUTELY ESSENTIAL GUIDE TO LONDON	David Benedictus	£4.95 ☐

All Sphere books are available at your local bookshop or newsagent, or can be ordered direct from the publisher. Just tick the titles you want and fill in the form below.

Name _____

Address _____

_____

Write to Sphere Books, Cash Sales Department, P.O. Box 11, Falmouth, Cornwall TR10 9EN

Please enclose a cheque or postal order to the value of the cover price plus:

UK: 55p for the first book, 22p for the second book and 14p for each additional book ordered to a maximum charge of £1.75.

OVERSEAS: £1.00 for the first book plus 25p per copy for each additional book.

BFPO & EIRE: 55p for the first book, 22p for the second book plus 14p per copy for the next 7 books, thereafter 8p per book.

Sphere Books reserve the right to show new retail prices on covers which may differ from those previously advertised in the text or elsewhere, and to increase postal rates in accordance with the PO.